WOMEN'S WORK
IS NEVER DONE

WOMEN'S WORK IS NEVER DONE

COMPARATIVE STUDIES IN CAREGIVING, EMPLOYMENT, AND SOCIAL POLICY REFORM

Edited by
Sylvia Bashevkin

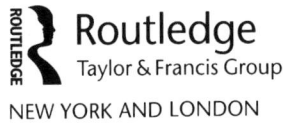

Routledge
Taylor & Francis Group
NEW YORK AND LONDON

Published in 2002 by
Routledge
711 Third Avenue
New York, NY 10017, USA

Published in Great Britain by
Routledge
2 Park Square, Milton Park
Abingdon, Oxon OX14 4RN

Routledge is an imprint of the Taylor & Francis Group, an informa business

Copyright © 2002 by Taylor & Francis Books, Inc.

Design and typography: Jack Donner

All rights reserved. No part of this book may be reprinted or reproduced or utilized in any form or by any electronic, mechanical, or other means, now known or hereafter invented, including photocopying and recording, or in any information storage or retrieval system, without permission in writing from the publishers.

Library of Congress Cataloging-in-Publication data

Women's work is never done : comparative studies in care-giving, employment, and social policy reform / edited by Sylvia Bashevkin.
    p. cm.
  Includes bibliographical references and index.
  ISBN 0-415-93480-X (hardback) — ISBN 0-415-93481-8 (pbk.)
  1. Women—Government policy—Cross-cultural studies. 2. Caregivers—Cross-cultural studies. 3. Sexual division of labor—Cross-cultural studies.
4. Welfare state—Cross-cultural studies. I. Title: Comparative studies in care-giving,
  employment, and social policy reform. II. Bashevkin, Sylvia B.

HQ1236 .W656 2002
305.42—dc21

2002023010

Contents

Acknowledgments vii

Introduction 1
Sylvia Bashevkin

Part I Conceptual Issues

1. **Normative Concepts in Dutch Policies on Work and Care** 15
   Selma Sevenhuijsen

Part II Confronting Women's Diversity

2. **It's No Longer Just about Race** 41
   Social Constructions of American Citizenship in the Moynihan Report
   Dionne Bensonsmith

3. **Paying for Caring** 67
   The Gendering Consequences of European Care Allowances
   for the Frail Elderly
   Jane Jenson

Part III Anglo-American Welfare Reform

4. **Poverty, Social Assistance, and the Employability** 85
   of Mothers in Four Commonwealth Countries
   Maureen Baker

5. **Road-Testing the Third Way** 113
   Single Mothers and Welfare Reform during the Clinton, Chrétien,
   and Blair Years
   Sylvia Bashevkin

Part IV Policy Alternatives

6. **Violating Women** 141
   Rights Abuses in the American Welfare Police State
   Gwendolyn Mink

7. **Mandatory "Marriage" or Obligatory Waged Work** 165
   Social Assistance and Single Mothers in Wisconsin and Ontario
   Leah F. Vosko

Contributors 201

Index 203

Acknowledgments

Unlike many other books, this collection began as a twinkle in an editor's eye at a scholarly conference. Karen Wolny, at the time with Palgrave/ St. Martin's and now publishing director at Routledge, attended a women and the welfare state panel at the International Political Science Association meetings in Quebec City in the summer of 2000. Maureen Baker, Gwendolyn Mink, Leah F. Vosko, and I presented papers, and Sandra Burt, of the Department of Political Science at the University of Waterloo in Waterloo, Ontario, Canada, served as the discussant. Karen's belief that our four manuscripts should be brought together in a larger, book-length collection led me to seek out Selma Sevenhuijsen, who presented her paper at another IPSA session, as well as Dionne Bensonsmith and Jane Jenson, who participated in panels at the American Political Science Association meetings in Washington, D.C., later that same summer.

All seven of us revised our papers in the fall of 2000, after which I submitted them together with an introductory chapter. My ability to work on this project was assisted by a six-month sabbatical leave in fall term 2000, secured for me by Robert Vipond as chair of the Department of Political Science at the University of Toronto. The refereeing process produced many valuable suggestions for improving the manuscript, as did a one-day book workshop in May 2001 with four University of Toronto political science Ph.D. students, Gina Cosentino, Genevieve Johnson, Jacqueline Krikorian, and Heather Murray. Nanda Purandare provided invaluable research assistance at the copyediting stage.

I am thankful to all of the chapter authors, editors, and commentators who have played such a pivotal role in creating and improving the various parts of this book. Funding from the Social Sciences and Humanities Research Council of Canada made it possible for me to attend the IPSA and APSA conferences and to convene the book workshop in Toronto. Above all, my family provided the encouragement necessary to keep the project interesting, relevant, and on track.

Sylvia Bashevkin
Toronto
September 2001

Introduction

Sylvia Bashevkin

Do contemporary Anglo-American and West European welfare states show more signs of resilience or decline? Do patterns of policy talk and policy change in these systems reflect more cross-national similarities than differences, more points of convergence than divergence? How have recent shifts in North American and European social policies affected different groups of women citizens? In what ways do unpaid caregiving and paid (including caregiving) employment intersect in the lives of female citizens?

These questions and others like them follow from two distinct streams of scholarly literature that address welfare state development in advanced industrial countries. Influential accounts of welfare regime formation, notably by Gøsta Esping-Andersen, and of contemporary regime restructuring, including by Paul Pierson, raise fundamental questions about convergence, resilience, and the role of states and markets in constructing, as well as refashioning, social policy schemes.[1] Like other mainstream studies in this field, these accounts tend to overlook women's crucial status, both as the main adult recipients of postwar income support benefits and as the primary providers of paid and unpaid care in modern welfare systems.

A second body of literature, which presents feminist perspectives on welfare states, has emerged since the 1970s to interrogate and expand the traditional base of knowledge in this field. Beginning with classic studies such as Barbara Nelson's analysis of the early two-channel welfare state in the United States, robust for employed men (via unemployment insurance) but residual for widowed women (under mothers' pensions), feminist scholarship has employed a gender lens to shed light on significant dimensions of social policy evolution that were missed by conventional analysts.[2] One popular focus of feminist research attention has been Esping-Andersen's typology of welfare regimes and, in particular, his account of the role of state programs in "decommodification," meaning the purposive release of citizens from reliance on labor market income. By addressing the varied uses of social benefits to cushion against the loss of earned income, Esping-Andersen theorized welfare state regimes in terms of two key units—states and markets. His conceptual approach thus turned on the extent to which states protected citizens, using decommodifying social programs, from labor market failures.

Feminist students of welfare state programs have closely scrutinized Esping-Andersen's typology, which contrasts liberal, residual, and predominantly Anglo-American welfare regimes with more generous, market-usurping (or decommodifying), and primarily continental European corporatist and social democratic ones. If any core conclusions can be said to emerge from this growing critical literature, they are at least three in number. First, traditional scholarly preoccupations with the relative significance of states and markets have obscured the differential relations of women and men to these core units of analysis, including within countries. Governments have operated in varied, and profoundly gendered, ways vis-à-vis their citizens, as have unfettered, regulated, and state-controlled markets. Organized interests that work to identify and challenge these patterns of differentiation—notably, women's movements—are frequently overlooked in welfare state studies that emphasize the role of trade union organizations, which were themselves traditionally male-dominated in most countries.

Second, feminist studies propose that an additional pillar, the family, be added to the state/market nexus. Given the fundamental importance of family units to constructions of society and hence social policy formation, it seems difficult to understand welfare state developments without addressing this dimension. In particular, scholars working in a critical feminist stream argue that the ability of women to create and maintain autonomous households represents a meaningful and gender-sensitive measure to distinguish among state/market/family regimes. Third, many feminist studies emphasize the impact of not just policy action but also policy talk or discourse, particularly as it frames discussions of "dependence," "personal responsibility," and women's roles within households.[3]

This volume draws together a provocative set of studies within the feminist welfare state stream; as a group, they offer a mixture of normative and empirical perspectives. All were initially presented as scholarly papers at conferences in the summer of 2000, either at the International Political Science Association meetings in Quebec City, Canada, or at the American Political Science Association meetings in Washington, D.C. Taken as a group, they help to define the contours of a second-generation literature about women and the welfare state that evaluates in a comparative way both the policy and discursive dimensions of state/market/family relations.

The purpose of the collection is to illuminate far more than simply the limitations of mainstream studies. Rather, its goal is to pursue the retrenchment and dismantlement issues raised by Pierson and others, with particular reference to women in Anglo-American and continental European welfare states. Using an analytic lens that focuses on differential impacts of social policy changes among women, we ask how developments at the levels of discourse, as well as action, have influenced caring responsibilities, paid employment, and women's status as citizens. By casting a wide net that includes scholars who have studied and experienced contemporary changes in the United States, Canada, and other Anglo-American systems, as well as in the Netherlands and other continental European cases, we offer a richly comparative perspective that would be absent if the collection focused exclusively on any one country or continent.

This volume breaks new ground in a number of respects with reference to the feminist social policy literature. At one level, it rejects assumptions about the fixed or static nature of welfare regimes by focusing explicitly on change over time in a given country or group of countries. Chapter authors frequently direct their attention toward dynamic questions of social policy resilience or decline, rather than toward older concerns about the utility of Esping-Andersen's typology for research on women and welfare states.⁴ Next, they work to elucidate the differential effects of shifts in policy talk and policy action among varied groups of women. Rather than reinforcing the prevailing focus in the literature on male/female variations in welfare state outcomes, this collection tries to move the pivot toward female/ female variations, including along the lines of race in the United States (chapter 2) and age in Western Europe (chapter 3).

As well, in its explicit focus on issues facing women as caregivers and care-receivers, the collection tries to push beyond existing treatments of females as either paid workers facing a variety of household, as well as labor market, obstacles or potentially autonomous citizens who are impeded by various familial obligations.⁵ Finally, the studies included in this volume contribute to a number of debates about women's citizenship status in advanced industrial countries. Some probe the fate, in times of neoliberal economic restructuring, of T. H. Marshall's concept of an expansive and universal social citizenship.⁶ Others ask how the demands of caregiving and paid employment intersect in the lives of low-income single mothers, especially as welfare states retrench and press a traditional, patriarchal view of family organization.⁷ Citizenship is thus approached at a number of different levels, including as a social and discursive construction and as a set of institutional arrangements that alternately confers or constrains far more than simple legal notions of "who is a citizen."

The book is divided into four subsections, to assist readers in thinking about conceptual, women's diversity, cross-national, and policy alternative questions. The text opens with an overview of major conceptual issues in the field of caregiving, employment, and social policy. In chapter 1, Selma Sevenhuijsen introduces an ethic of care lens to evaluate contemporary government documents from the Netherlands, a country in which state-funded public allowances were created to subsidize carers' work. Sevenhuijsen grapples with the normative consequences of such payments, asking how they affected women as citizens, workers, and members of families. Her examination of the Dutch case also sheds light on international spillover effects in the social policy field—notably, the growing influence in the Netherlands of Anglo-American notions of economic self-reliance and self-sufficiency.

According to Sevenhuijsen, the concept of care speaks directly to notions of interdependence and relational autonomy in civil society, where citizens "need each other in order to live a good life." Yet many of the Dutch government documents she examines were grounded in an approach that contrasted independence with dependence and that framed caring activities as obstacles to independence. Sevenhuijsen argues that independence needs to be reconceived in more socially interdependent terms, perhaps as "the capacity to find a balance between care for the self, care for others, and care for the world." This revised view helps to place questions about caring at the center of ongoing debates about state/market/family relations; as well, it challenges older assumptions in the feminist literature to the effect that the primary goal of policy reform is to make individual women more autonomous vis-à-vis the market and family. Moreover, Sevenhuijsen's formulation helps to contrast ideas about social interdependence, on one side, with neoliberal emphases on unencumbered, independent, and "personally responsible" individuals, on the other.

The second part of the volume considers how changes in welfare state regimes have affected diverse subgroups of women within Western industrialized countries. In chapter 2, Dionne Bensonsmith addresses racial divisions in the United States. Her examination focuses on the Moynihan Report, a controversial 1965 document prepared by Daniel Patrick Moynihan when he served in the Johnson administration. Bensonsmith pays close attention to the Moynihan Report's discussion of what it termed "the deterioration of the Negro family."[8] She argues that this document helped not only to institutionalize stereotypic views of African-American women, but also to define sex roles in this minority community according to a simplistic male breadwinner/provider versus female nurturer/dependent dichotomy. Over time, Bensonsmith contends, the Moynihan Report contributed to a highly racialized understanding of the rights and obligations of citizenship in the United States. Moreover, she argues, it assisted in the creation of a racially biased discursive as well as policy context, in which welfare debates continue to unfold through the early twenty-first century.

Parallel with Selma Sevenhuijsen's discussion in chapter 1,

Dionne Bensonsmith's contribution in chapter 2 rejects older binary divisions grounded in male/female, public/private, and independence/dependence dichotomies. Both authors base their critiques of these models on a close reading of official government documents: Sevenhuijsen draws on reports about caring in the Netherlands, while Bensonsmith examines a very influential study of African-American families. Bensonsmith's chapter demonstrates how race, gender, and class intersected in social constructions of citizenship in the United States dating back to the 1960s. In her words, the discourse of the Moynihan Report helped to implant notions that African-American women were impaired citizens, since they were portrayed as either "emasculating black matriarchs" or "fertile and lazy welfare queens."

Jane Jenson's discussion in chapter 3 of public allowances for frail seniors shines a spotlight on age-based diversity in West European welfare states. Women constitute a large proportion not only of the elderly who require care, but also of the people who provide their care. Jenson assesses the variations in care allowance schemes that developed across Western Europe and concludes that many shifted over time from state or public schemes toward increasingly market-based arrangements that ostensibly offered more "choice" to consumers. In her view, care allowances based on ideas of market "choice" were unlikely to alter traditional gender relations in these established welfare states, in part because care payments rarely provided secure, full-time, well-paid employment for the women who performed such work. They could, however, offer greater economic security to the elderly women who received such allowances than was available in the past. In other words, public allowances might entrench some measure of autonomy for the frail seniors who received them, at the same time as they did little to revalue the labor of younger women who performed the caring work.

Jenson's account is particularly important because it links contentious policy questions about home care and seniors' allowances with broader conceptual issues of citizenship and diversity among women. In her view, shifts in the direction of "choice"-based care arrangements only reinforced a larger trend toward privileging market relations in Western Europe and other advanced industrial systems. Values associated with second-wave women's movements, notably gender equality, became overshadowed by this focus on market options. According to Jenson, the elevation of economic norms had a direct effect on the ability of working-age women to earn their way within the labor markets of Western Europe. Her research suggests that marketized care allowance schemes for frail seniors—most of them female—directly threatened the labor force circumstances and hence economic autonomy of women who worked as carers.

The third part of this collection explores welfare state changes across a variety of Anglo-American contexts. Chapter 4 by Maureen Baker addresses social assistance reform and women's employment in four Commonwealth countries: Australia, Canada, Great Britain, and New Zealand. Baker contends that single mothers on social assistance benefits faced diverse consequences as a result of neoliberal economic restructuring initiatives in these systems. She shows, for example, that lone mothers were required to pursue paid employment when their youngest child was six months old in one province in Canada, while the comparable age in Australia remained sixteen years. Baker links cross-national variations in employability rules to a number of factors, including rates of female paid labor force participation, where levels in Canada paralleled those in the United States and exceeded those in the other three cases, and cultural assumptions about women's caregiving and men's breadwinning roles, where Australians tended toward traditional values.

Baker's discussion carries through with the theme of diversity from part II of this volume and extends that focus to differences in employability policies across seemingly similar Anglo-American democracies. Her study demonstrates a pattern whereby relatively high overall rates of female participation in the full-time paid labor force (notably in Canada) were associated with greater policy attention to child-care issues, higher divorce rates, lower fertility rates, and more pronounced efforts to press lone mothers into paid employment. Baker's ability to trace variations across four Commonwealth countries on these kinds of measures underlines the differential responses of similar systems to ongoing pressures for economic restructuring.

In chapter 5, Sylvia Bashevkin compares social policy developments during three "post-conservative" or Third Way political executives: President Bill Clinton in the United States, Prime Minister Jean Chrétien in Canada, and Prime Minister Tony Blair in Britain. Bashevkin argues that welfare state changes under their watch included the introduction of an expanded layer of work-tested social benefits on top of existing means-tested ones, along with shifts in the direction of both tax-based or fiscalized social policy and an increasingly compromised or threadbare notion of social citizenship. She suggests that even though the public discourse of Clinton, Chrétien, and Blair seemed muted, reasonable, and balanced, particularly when compared with that of their predecessors, the Third Way policies they pursued could produce a more radically conservative restructuring of welfare regimes than was undertaken by the Republican and Tory political executives who preceded them.

Parallel with Baker's approach in chapter 4, Bashevkin's study uses a similar case methodology to explore patterns of convergence and divergence in Anglo-American welfare policy. She shows how the United States during the Clinton years advanced further down the path of work-tested benefits, taxified social policy, and eroded or compromised social citizenship than did Canada under Chrétien or Britain under Blair. As well, Bashevkin's chapter illuminates the discursive dimension of Third Way developments in probing the use of "personal responsibility" rhetoric by these leaders. In her view, rather than asserting a structural or material approach to what was once called poverty, Clinton, Chrétien, and Blair reinforced a moralistic view—championed by their predecessors, including Ronald Reagan and Margaret Thatcher—of the individual behavioral failings of lone mothers.

The fourth section of the collection considers policy alternatives presently on offer in North American systems. In chapter 6, Gwendolyn Mink assesses the impact of the 1996 Personal Responsibility and Work Opportunity Reconciliation Act (PRWORA) in the United States. According to Mink, this legislation established an extremely punitive regime predicated on compromising the vocational freedom, sexual privacy, and reproductive choices of low-income women. As well, the damage done by PRWORA was compounded by a series of "fathers' rights" initiatives in the U.S. Congress that pressed hard on the presumed virtues of marriage and father-headed families. As an alternative to PRWORA and "fathers' rights" approaches, Mink endorses the creation of a caregivers' income system in the United States; in her view, such a scheme would help to challenge racialized assumptions about the lack of socially valuable work performed by poor women who care for their children.

Gwendolyn Mink's examination of the consequences of PRWORA fits closely with Sylvia Bashevkin's discussion in the previous chapter of ideational change under Third Way leaders. Mink's argument reinforces Bashevkin's claim that moralistic approaches to social policy had measurable effects; in the U.S. case, one clear upshot was the creation of what Mink describes as a federally sanctioned "welfare police state." Her discussion also dovetails closely with Selma Sevenhuijsen's critique in chapter 1 of "dependency" and "choice" rhetoric and with Jane Jenson's assessment in chapter 3 of care allowance policies. Mink's contribution is particularly important in its effort to propose a European-style paid caring approach in the United States, as one alternative to PRWORA and fathers' rights initiatives.

In chapter 7, Leah F. Vosko examines social assistance reform in two subnational jurisdictions, Wisconsin in the United States and Ontario in Canada. Vosko evaluates workfare-style programs in both places in light of federal policy changes effected in 1996, which created increasingly decentralized, residual, and work-oriented social policy regimes in the United States and Canada. Over time, single mothers in jurisdictions like Wisconsin and Ontario faced a narrowing set of choices between what Vosko terms "mandatory marriage or obligatory waged work." Her chapter addresses the question of caregiving allowances as an alternative to punitive workfare regimes and offers a more critical assessment of this proposal than does Gwendolyn Mink in chapter 6.

Vosko's analysis compares two subnational units in North America, showing how pressures to reduce federal welfare spending and devolve greater power to states and provinces produced similar workfare schemes on both sides of the 49th parallel. Although the specific terms of W-2 in Wisconsin and Ontario Works in Canada varied, both regimes left single mothers with few alternatives other than attaching to a man or complying with mandatory work-for-welfare schemes. In an effort to transcend these two options, Vosko devotes attention at the end of her chapter to assessing the advantages and disadvantages of care allowances, parental leave programs, and universal child-care schemes. Echoing Sevenhuijsen's opening chapter, Vosko concludes that research on welfare reform needs to consider work and care issues in tandem, rather than as dichotomous units.

Taken together, these chapters provide an unusually comparative and dynamic look at key questions of welfare state research. They trace the treatment of caring, paid employment, and social citizenship at normative and discursive levels, including in the highly racialized environment of the United States and in the increasingly age-stratified societies of Western Europe. The authors probe what neoliberal restructuring strategies have meant to the sexual, familial, and employment lives of poor women, especially in residual Anglo-American cases like the United States, Canada, and Britain. They evaluate the strengths and weaknesses of European-style care allowances as an alternative to dominant social assistance reform directions, including mandatory work-for-welfare, thus contributing to ongoing North American debates over policy alternatives.

It is difficult to draw neat conclusions from any collection of articles that examines so many different countries, each with varied approaches to social policy. Yet in general terms, it seems fair to report that the welfare states considered in this book were far less resilient—or less robust, in programmatic terms—than a reading of the conventional literature on policy retrenchment would indicate.[9] Moreover, these regimes as a group appeared to use increasingly market-based, work-oriented, and moralistic approaches to their women citizens, a cross-national parallel that is far from obvious in the mainstream literature. By emphasizing the language, as well as actions, of government elites and by providing an explicitly cross-national look at women's experiences of welfare state transformation, the present collection serves to illuminate our understanding of caregiving, employment, and social policy reform. Above all, it encourages future analysts to probe further the terms under which the social citizenship of varied groups of women is contested and arguably endangered in an age of welfare retrenchment.

Notes

1. See Gøsta Esping-Andersen, *Politics against Markets: The Social Democratic Road to Power* (Princeton: Princeton University Press, 1985); Gøsta Esping-Andersen, *The Three Worlds of Welfare Capitalism* (Princeton: Princeton University Press, 1990); and Paul Pierson, *Dismantling the Welfare State? Reagan, Thatcher, and the Politics of Retrenchment* (Cambridge: Cambridge University Press, 1994).
2. See Barbara J. Nelson, "The Origins of the Two-Channel Welfare State: Workmen's Compensation and Mothers' Aid," in *Women, the State, and Welfare*, ed. Linda Gordon (Madison: University of Wisconsin Press, 1990), 123–51.
3. A number of other edited volumes and monographs have been published in this field. For comparative critiques of the established literature, see Diane Sainsbury, ed., *Gendering Welfare States* (London: Sage, 1994); Diane Sainsbury, *Gender, Equality, and Welfare States* (Cambridge: Cambridge University Press, 1996); Diane Sainsbury, ed., *Gender and Welfare State Regimes* (Oxford: Oxford University Press, 1999); Julia S. O'Connor, Ann Shola Orloff, and Sheila Shaver, *States, Markets, Families: Gender, Liberalism, and Social Policy in Australia, Canada, Great Britain, and the United States* (Cambridge: Cambridge University Press, 1999); and Mary Daly, *The Gender Division of Welfare: The Impact of the British and German Welfare States* (Cambridge: Cambridge University Press, 2000).

   On discursive issues, see Wendy Sarvasy, "Reagan and Low-Income Mothers: A Feminist Recasting of the Debate," in *Remaking the Welfare State: Retrenchment and Social Policy in America and Europe*, ed. Michael K. Brown (Philadelphia: Temple University Press, 1988), 253–76; Martha Ackelsberg, "Feminist Analyses of Public Policy," *Comparative Politics* 24 (1992): 486, 490; Nancy Fraser and Linda Gordon, "'Dependency' Demystified: Inscriptions of Power in a Keyword of the Welfare State," *Social Politics* 1 (1994): 4–31; Ricky Solinger, "Dependency and Choice: The Two Faces of Eve," in *Whose Welfare?*, ed. Gwendolyn Mink (Ithaca, N.Y.: Cornell University Press, 1999), 7–35; and Eva Feder Kittay, "Welfare, Dependency, and a Public Ethic of Care," in *Whose Welfare?*, ed. Mink, 189–213.
4. "Fit" with the Esping-Andersen typology constituted a major preoccupation of previous efforts in this field. See, for example, Sainsbury, ed., *Gendering Welfare States*.

5. For one example of a predominantly male/female conceptual focus with an emphasis on autonomous individuals, see O'Connor et al., *States, Markets, Families*.
6. See T. H. Marshall, "Citizenship and Social Class," in T. H. Marshall and Tom Bottomore, *Citizenship and Social Class* (London: Pluto, 1992). This focus is particularly clear in chapters 3 and 5 of this volume by Jane Jenson and Sylvia Bashevkin, respectively.
7. Chapters 6 and 7 of this volume by Gwendolyn Mink and Leah F. Vosko, respectively, pay close attention to this issue.
8. Office of Policy Planning and Research, United States Department of Labor, *The Negro Family: The Case for National Action*, March 1965, 5.
9. See Pierson, *Dismantling the Welfare State*; and Sylvia Bashevkin, "Rethinking Retrenchment: North American Social Policy during the Early Clinton and Chrétien Years," *Canadian Journal of Political Science* 33 (2000): 7–36.

Part I

Conceptual Issues

1.
Normative Concepts in Dutch Policies on Work and Care

Selma Sevenhuijsen

Introduction

Since 1995, the Dutch government has been engaged in developing an innovative policy program on work and care. That year, a special advisory committee proposed using a "combination scenario" as the goal for government policies. By acknowledging that caring labor had generally fallen on the shoulders of women, this proposal aimed to promote two forms of balance: first, a balance between men and women in paid work and care; and second, a balance between the use of paid and unpaid care. The combination approach was noteworthy because it moderated the exclusive focus on the integration of women in paid labor that had dominated older equal opportunity policies.

This chapter presents a normative analysis of the Dutch government report on the combination scenario and related policy documents, using the ethic of care as a lens for analysis and evaluation.[1] The combination scenario has created space in public policy-making for a more thorough appraisal of care and offers opportunities for developing new forms of policy-making in this field. At the same time, however, a full appraisal of care is hampered by the terms of the distributive policy paradigm that created this space, in which care is overwhelmingly conceptualized as unpaid work. By thinking in terms of a dichotomy between work and care and by positioning care in a separate life sphere, this paradigm not only tends to reproduce the public/private divide, but also overlooks the moral complexities of caring practices and the transformational potential of care as a political concept. It is my contention that a feminist ethic of care can help to bypass these problems, particularly if we conceptualize care as a citizenship concept.

In order to introduce my argument, I first present a normative analysis of some of the main policy documents. What are the goals of the proposed policies? How is care conceptualized in them? What are the leading normative concepts? The conceptual problems associated with the policy framework can then be identified. In the second section, I elaborate on some of the characteristics of care ethics that together provide alternative starting points for thinking about the place of care in the proposed policies. In the third section, I propose a reformulation of the normative concepts for work and care policies.

The Power of the Distributive Paradigm

The conceptual parameters of the current policy discussion were established during the 1980s, when the Dutch government drafted a new plan on emancipation calling for equal opportunity policies.[2] The plan maintained that the institutionalization of sexual difference was one of society's organizing principles, so that women not only systematically confronted barriers in their development, but also were held back in public and private life. According to this report, unequal power relations between men and women were revealed not only in the prevailing division of human labor, but also in the normalization of intimate relations and sexuality. Creating more independence for women could alleviate their dependency on men, so that women would be guaranteed realistic possibilities for free choice.

Following on this problem definition, the 1985 policy plan stated that "every adult must have the opportunity to provide for and take care of themselves."[3] The emancipation policy's official goal was, then, formulated as follows: "Transforming current society, in which sexual difference is strongly institutionalized, to a pluriform society, where everybody, regardless of sex or civil status, has the possibility of achieving an independent existence, and in which women and men can realize equal rights, opportunities, liberties, and responsibilities."[4] The plan considered sharing the responsibility for domestic labor and the upbringing of children between men and women as important. At the same time, however, domestic arrangements were defined as a private responsibility; according to the report, the state ought to refrain from "prescribing to people how to live their lives." How the division of labor and care was organized would be determined by "individual choices for the arrangements of one's existence," choices that the report's authors believed government ought to respect.

This conceptual approach was maintained in subsequent years. At the same time, policy makers increasingly acknowledged the claim made by women's organizations that something needed to be done about the division of work in the home. In 1992, the Dutch coalition government formed by the Social Democrats and Christian Democrats decided to adopt three new so-called lines of action, one of which was the redistribution of unpaid work between men and women, so as to extend men's caring responsibility. The official policy goal remained, however, untouched. Emphasis continued to be placed on the integration of women in the labor market. A fairer division of household chores was introduced as a precondition for this to be achieved. The next government, a coalition between the Social Democrats and Liberals, retained a labor market approach to emancipation, since it fit with that regime's view that paid labor was the crucial means of achieving social integration.

The government committee on the division of unpaid work, which began its work in 1994, extended the redistributive approach to care/work.[5] Its task was to elaborate four possible future scenarios for the division of unpaid care versus paid work between men and women, and for the ratio of paid to unpaid care-work, and to select the best scenario from among them. The committee employed a macroeconomic approach to the issue of care, using large-scale studies of hours spent on various tasks by the Dutch population in the two preceding decades as its main source of empirical data. The goal was to explore the possible consequences of the four scenarios in terms of different forms of policy, in order to "influence the public and policy agenda."[6]

The report selected the so-called combination scenario. In this model, the total volume of paid care would increase until it equaled that of unpaid care. In the sphere of unpaid care, an equal division between men and women would be the goal, with the proviso that they must have the possibility to determine for themselves what they want to emphasize in different stages of their lives.[7] The concrete measures proposed by members of the committee, including the legal right to part-time labor, legal regulations for flexible working hours, enhanced child-care facilities, and different forms of caring leave, as well as a further individualization of social security and the fiscal system, all corresponded with their macroeconomic perspective.

This same outlook was revealed in the committee's view that the two-earner household can best be encouraged by such financial measures as abolishing the tax bonus for breadwinners. The tax bonus abolition argument is based on a neoclassical stimulus–response model that assumes individuals are mainly motivated by financial considerations in their life choices. Overall, the normative framework of the report can be characterized as a mixture of neoclassical economic assumptions about human nature and social life, with a liberal political framework about the ideal relationship between the state and its citizens. Together, these elements can be said to form the basis of the so-called distributive paradigm.[8]

In spite of the fact that care was its primary focus, the report translated all aspects of care into the terminology of unpaid and paid work, time spending, citizens' preferences, and choice. However, throughout the text there appeared elements of an alternative appraisal of care. In its overview of then-current government policies, for example, the committee stated that the growing political attention devoted to caring labor should be seen as "an overture for future policy in which care would have to acquire an independent place, regardless of work."[9] Furthermore, in the concluding chapter, the committee noted that its qualitative judgment about the different scenarios was grounded in a view that the preferred scenario should be in keeping with the "culture concerning the care of children and the aged." Without further reference or qualification, it proposed that "for reasons of quality of care and upbringing, the Dutch prefer to partially care for themselves."[10]

The Search for a Definition of Care

In 1996, the Dutch Emancipation Council recommended to the government a new concept in social security law, to guide future policies. The idea of "care independence," which resembles the English concept of self-reliance, suggested "that everybody should be responsible and independent in three spheres of life: that of care, that of labor and income, and that of leisure and social life. Women and men can only attain independence in these different spheres when responsibilities are shared in a new way."[11]

In this statement, care is once again confined to a separate sphere. Independence remains the hegemonic norm and care is simply tagged onto it. This same approach can also be seen in the normative framework proposed by the Emancipation Council for the life sphere of care: "Care independence and responsibility in the life sphere of care: every adult individual has the opportunity of caring for themselves, for their own life context and for care dependents (those who are not or no longer capable of caring for themselves)."[12] Again, "self-care" is taken as the norm. This "self-caring" individual becomes the prototypical representation of the normal citizen in all of the Council's policy texts. This normative citizen apparently does not need to be cared for by others. Care-receivers are represented as a separate group; they figure as the objects of care by the "care independents." Independence and self-sufficiency are thus preserved as the core values of emancipated citizenship.

In 1996, the Dutch government also introduced a new white paper to guide future emancipation policies. This document reflected on whether the new policies remained consistent with the official goals of 1985 and their three normative principles: pluriformity, independence, and equal rights. According to the 1996 document, pluriformity accorded with an emphasis on social diversity, but could be at odds with the norm of equality if the latter were treated as equality of results or outcomes. Conversely, if equality were defined as equality of opportunity or starting positions, then it could be combined with pluriformity. Equality, therefore, can best be regarded as a precondition for independence and pluriformity.

Once again, independence figured as the single overarching norm of the 1996 document. This was revealed in the government's subsequent reaction to critics who claimed that independence was too narrowly confined to economic independence and that "other forms like care independence have been made subservient to this."[13] According to government rebuttals, this one-sidedness can be overcome by adopting a distinction among three life spheres as proposed by the Emancipation Council and by regarding all three as equal in value, each with its own independence norm. The personal life sphere should be guided by care independence, the labor and income sphere by economic independence, and the sociopolitical sphere by independent judgment and social self-reliance. These ideas also permitted the government to introduce arguments about responsibility in its discourse, which stated that independence and responsibility were unevenly shared between men and women. Women bore greater responsibility for caring, while men viewed their primary responsibility as a financial one.[14]

In a passage explicitly about care, the white paper employed several different definitions. At one point, it argued that the representation and appraisal of care should be improved for new policies to be successful. This concerned not only the care of children, but also the care of family members and "other relations" so that men would regard it as self-evident that they needed to participate in care. The paper also introduced a broader concept of care, in arguing that notions like equality and independence were usually linked with the individual. Yet individualized ideas should change, since "regarding modern emancipated relationships, society pays more attention to social relations and to the question of mutual care and responsibility."[15] Social responsibility thus stretches beyond the relationships in the nuclear family. It includes voluntary labor and informal care for relatives outside the direct family. The conclusion is that the government will, alongside equality and independence, also pay attention to social responsibility and "care in a wider sense."[16]

A subsequent government white paper titled "Towards a New Balance between Work and Care," published in 1999, opened by stating its preference for a broad and somewhat vaguely defined concept of care:

it is not only the combination of paid labor with caring for the family or others, but also adequate time for one's own development, education or other social activities. Men and women should have the opportunity of choosing paid labor in combination with other responsibilities, without it leading to an unacceptable work pressure or an over organized existence.[17]

Once again, an economic vocabulary set the tone of the discussion, since stress and burnout were presented as dangers that justified the proposed policies. Furthermore, care itself was not elaborated upon, since nowhere was the activity of caring actually defined. Just as significant was the white paper's presentation of care solely from the perspective of the caregivers, the persons with the double load, and caring was confined to looking after family members. The relational perspective on care, as announced in the 1996 document, was not elaborated on. This is not surprising, since by 1999, the government had decided to preserve the individualistic goals of the 1985 emancipation policies, rather than to embrace the more collectivist orientation of earlier initiatives.

Problems with the Distributive Paradigm

The distributive paradigm is permeated with interlocking dualisms, the most conspicuous of which are independence and dependence, caregiving and care-receiving, and public and private. Caring for others is continually perceived as a barrier to independence, while dependence has negative connotations, in that it is perceived as an impediment to independent citizenship. A discursive opposition is thus produced between independent and dependent citizens, so that vulnerability and hence the need for care are projected onto specific groups who are stigmatized as "dependent." Care is thus equated with protection.

Despite the professed desires of the Dutch government to bring about a better balance between "paid and unpaid care work," care gradually became confined to the so-called private sphere and turned into a private responsibility. This is paradoxical, since the 1999 Dutch government approach also sought to construct a more extensive sense of collective responsibility for care provision. The further development of this idea, however, was hampered by notions that the state should not intervene in its citizens' "lifestyle choices." The latter approach fails to acknowledge that the state *does* already construct the parameters of gendered social life by continuing to support the breadwinner/ caretaker model and by (re)constructing boundaries between public and private responsibilities.

As well, the distributive paradigm's individualistic assumptions (visible both in its image of human nature and in its guiding normative principles) remain barriers to recognizing the relational dimensions of care. They ignore the fact that care not only is about the provision of physical, material, and educational needs, but it also operates as a medium to shape relationships, connections, and commitment; to transfer culture; and to contribute on a daily basis to the meaning of human existence. The passage in the scenario report on Dutch culture, which has been quoted in nearly every policy document on this issue, contains some rather confused thoughts about the meaning of culture. First, it homogenizes culture, as if there were no within-country differences in the Netherlands. Second, it turns culture into a static phenomenon that remains constant throughout the years. And third, it is built on the idea that care cultures are an external factor to policies, as if they were not heavily influenced by public decisions.

These flaws are related to a larger problem—namely, the inability to define care in an encompassing manner. The work approach to care has had the undeniable advantage of bringing issues regarding the division of domestic labor and household chores to the attention of policy makers. Yet once these issues are framed in primarily neoclassical economic terms, as has been the usual practice, the discourse absorbs a built-in blind spot for the moral and relational dimensions of care.[18] It is therefore ironic that the acclaimed "reappraisal of care," dating from 1999, is expected to flow from factors external to the policy sphere itself. The desired change is expected first and foremost from men, who increasingly figure in official documents as the primary problem. It is difficult to imagine, then, that the need for reappraisal might rest in the labor market–oriented policy paradigm in the first place.

Injecting the Ethic of Care

The contribution that an ethic of care could make becomes apparent when we consider its alternative definition of care. The literature on this topic focuses on the complex intertwining of care as work and care as a moral orientation, in a context of attentiveness and commitment. This approach is encapsulated in the idea of care as a social practice and a social process.[19] The definition of care provided by Berenice Fisher and Joan Tronto provides a strong foundation for political argument: "On the most general level, we suggest that caring be viewed as a *species activity that includes everything we do to maintain, continue, and repair our 'world' so that we can live in it as well as possible*. That world includes our bodies, our selves, and our environment, all of which we seek to interweave in a complex, life-sustaining web."[20]

There are at least five reasons why this approach has the capacity to renew the policy discussion of work and care. First, it illustrates that care not only concerns "others," but that everybody has to reconcile care for others with care for the self on a daily basis. This idea diverges from the oppositions between self and other, and between independence and dependence, that underlie the distributive paradigm. The ethic of care definition is based on the assumption that everybody needs care and that everybody in principle has the ability to provide care. Furthermore, it makes clear that care concerns not only people, but also material things; by placing an emphasis on this connection, it becomes possible to see the giving and receiving of care as a dimension of the quality of life.

Second, the Tronto definition makes clear that because care is inherently a relational activity, then a relational vocabulary and a relational view of human nature are needed to describe and judge caring practices. Individuals usually live in complex networks of care, in which they sometimes provide care and sometimes receive it, often without noticing. The notion of interdependence provides a better starting point for arguing about care than does a dichotomous opposition between independence and dependence. In the ethic of care approach, dependence is not an inherently negative phenomenon. In many care situations, it is simply a fact of life, which poses complex moral dilemmas for the different actors involved. Instead, dependency has a double-edged relationship with power: Power relations create dependency and dependency creates power in its turn. When we take caring practices as a starting point in our argument, we can say that dealing with the triangle of dependency, power, and vulnerability is the core moral problematic for an ethic of care.[21]

Third, the definition makes clear that discussions about care must always distinguish between the caregivers' and the care-receivers' positions and perspectives. If "care" is used as a container concept, then the perspective from which it is discussed is silently subsumed under it. In order to clarify this, we can view care as Joan Tronto does, as an ongoing process consisting of different related phases or dimensions, each with a different value connected to it.[22] *Caring about* implies recognition that care is necessary: noting a need and making an assessment that this need should be met. The corresponding value is that of attentiveness. The second phase, *taking care of*, consists of assuming some responsibility for the identified need, determining how to respond to it, and taking steps to meet the need in question. The corresponding value is that of responsibility. *Caregiving* involves the direct meeting of needs for care. It involves physical work and almost always requires that caregivers come in contact with the objects of care. The corresponding value is competence: the development of expertise and the disposal of resources to carry out the caring acts. *Care-receiving* is the final phase. It recognizes that the object of care will respond to the care it receives. The corresponding value is that of responsiveness. This refers to the necessity of optimal interaction between caregiver and care-receiver about the nature of the need and the quality of the care.

According to Tronto, these four values of attentiveness, responsibility, competence, and responsiveness form the core of an ethic of care. If we regard dealing with the triangle of power, dependency, and vulnerability as the core moral problematic of an ethic of care, then we should add trust to this list, since it is a value that cuts through the different phases. When we take these ideas as a point of departure, it becomes clear that the crucial problem in the definitions of care in the official documents analyzed previously is that they focus exclusively on caregiving (the third phase), while singling it out from the rest of the caring process. By doing so, they also overlook the coherence and interdependence among the different dimensions of care.

The fourth advantage of the previous definition, then, is that it does not make care coincide with what is traditionally seen as "women's work," or caregiving in the private sphere of dependents. The definition enables one to discuss and determine who is or should be responsible for different locations of care and how the coordination between the different phases of care should be arranged. A broad definition of care cuts through the public/private divide and enables one to investigate how different responsibilities are defined and demarcated and how different actors in caring processes can cooperate. This underlines the need not only for a "combination scenario," but also for a "coordination scenario."[23]

Finally, this definition and the accompanying theoretical approach make it clear that caring practices have to be considered from the perspective of power and conflict. Too often, policy makers work from an implicit assumption that care stands surely for social harmony on a larger scale. This notion can probably be traced to hidden associations of care with femininity and unconditional love. It is more realistic to assume that care is both the object and the medium of power. The question of how needs are interpreted and assessed, who takes care of whom and under which conditions, directly concerns the division of resources and the capacity to invoke the care of others in order to lead a satisfying existence. Among caregivers, care-receivers, care-managers, and political decision makers, profound conflicting viewpoints often exist regarding the scale and quality of the care needed. Seen from the perspective of power, care is a double-edged sword: Care can be debilitating and patronizing, as well as enabling and supportive. We thus have to develop moral standards that enable us to evolve a democratic vision of care. Caring at its best is a responsible form of strategic acting. If we make care into a continuous topic of public deliberation, then it may be possible to formulate well-reflected values that can guide political judgment on this subject.

Reformulations

Against this background, I suggest, new values and normative concepts should become part of the Dutch debate on work and care, just as more familiar ideas should be reconsidered and redefined. I will first present some thoughts about new moral concepts and then turn to the more familiar ones. The values of attentiveness, responsibility, competence, responsiveness, and trust together provide a framework for a democratic processing of caring practices, both on an individual and a societal level. The meaning of these values is by no means self-evident. I will briefly indicate how they can be specified in the context of work and care.

Attentiveness implies a continual awareness of the need to care about human needs and human flourishing.[24] It implies active engagement in processes of needs interpretation in order to answer the question of what people require in order to lead satisfying lives. Attentiveness is not just a psychological disposition, despite the fact that the ability to be attentive is not inherent or developed by everybody. If we realize the extent of self-centeredness and willful ignorance in our culture, it becomes possible to see attentiveness as a moral achievement.[25] Attentiveness requires capacities like open-mindedness and careful listening as part of the democratic attitude.[26] It also assumes that citizens possess the ability to make distinctions between self and other, in order not to project their own needs onto others. Being attentive requires that one is attentive to one's own needs for care and can suspend one's own goals and concerns.[27] These thoughts may clarify why "care independence" is inadequate as a leading moral concept for a politics of care. It cannot capture the interrelational moral complexities implied in the first phase of caring.

Responsibility can best be conceptualized as the active willingness to take steps in order to ensure that something is to be done about the caring need. The corresponding moral question is, How can I best express my caring responsibility? Answers to this question are not simply bound to individuals; rather, they are the subject of extensive, conflict-ridden collective deliberations and moral practices. *Relationality* is again the catchword here. As the American moral philosopher Margaret Urban Walker states in her plea for an ethic of responsibility and integrity, "The basic claim about the structure of our responsibilities is this: Specific moral claims on us arise from our contact or relationship with others who are vulnerable to our actions and choices. We are *obligated to respond* to particular others when circumstance or ongoing relationship render them especially, conspicuously, or peculiarly dependent on us."[28]

In Walker's opinion, this demands a view of moral deliberation that is expressive, interpretative, and, where possible, collaborative. Moral deliberation thus conceived can deal with "moving horizons of commitments and adjustments" that are mediated by narratives of identity, relationship, and value.[29] Applied to the discussion of the combination of work and care, this approach permits a broader conceptualization of responsibility than is currently in play. In fact, the discussion itself can be seen as a moral practice of interpreting and assigning caring responsibilities. It should be emphasized that this view can be pursued fruitfully only when public debate aligns itself with social practices of dealing with caring responsibilities and when it is based on a thorough understanding of them. Otherwise, the public language of responsibility easily slips into a language of obligation that links care to duty ethics and is aimed at settling rights and duties in a top-down manner. The latter approach obscures two points: first, that the ethic of care does not easily fit into the vocabulary of duty ethics; and second, that it has a distinctive moral epistemology and image of human nature.[30]

The aim of understanding care as a moral practice of responsibility would also enhance the understanding of *competence*. In the context of care ethics, the value of competence refers to the need for caregivers to have the expertise, the time, and the material resources to do the concrete caring work as well as possible. One cannot fulfill a certain task or role if these are lacking. As Joan Tronto has argued, ensuring that caring work is done competently must be a moral aspect of care if the adequacy of the care given is to be a measure of its success.[31] This implies that decision makers should investigate what caregivers concretely need in terms of resources and social infrastructure in order to combine the different activities and responsibilities in their lives.

Responsiveness reflects most explicitly the fact that care is a shared practice, where the quality of the relationship between caregiver and care-receiver matters. Morally, it implies that the caregiver is open-minded toward the reactions of the care-receiver to the care received. This is important, since dealing with the triangle of dependency, vulnerability, and power is, as stated previously, the core moral question in caring practices. Given the very nature of dependency, caregivers have variable amounts of power vis-à-vis care-receivers. Politically, this points to the need to involve care-receivers in the new politics of care as much as possible, in order to evaluate whether the care conforms to their needs. Policies in the past have been overwhelmingly dominated by the caregivers' perspective. From the perspective of care as a social and moral practice, this is questionable, since it not only overlooks the relational dynamics of care, but also denies the fact that the needs and moral considerations of care-receivers should play a role in the new politics of care.

When we consider these values together, it becomes clear that they are indeed interdependent and intertwined. Adequate responsiveness requires attentiveness. Care can only proceed if people and institutions accept responsibility and provide or receive adequate resources so that care can be provided competently and effectively. This is clear when we see that responsiveness contains a dimension of communication, exchange, and reciprocity. As argued by Dutch legal philosopher Willem Witteveen, responsiveness implies active listening, replying, directly reacting to problems, and from there reaching decisions about what is to be done and how.[32] It implies accountability, or the willingness to publicly account for the reasons for and effects of one's actions.

As stated previously, *trust* can be seen as a link between these different values. The link between care and trust can be clarified according to Anette Baier's definition of trust. Trust, she says, is "letting other persons (or institutions like firms or nations) take care of something the truster cares about, where such 'caring for' involves some kind of discretionary power."[33] In her view, "trust is reliance on another's competence and willingness to look after, rather than harm things one cares about which are entrusted to the care-giver."[34] These statements encapsulate in a nutshell the four values of the ethic of care. For attentiveness to be effective, potential care-receivers must entrust their needs and their narratives about themselves to caregivers. If one entrusts something to somebody else, then the truster becomes dependent on the other's discernment, goodwill, and competence to take care of the entrusted goods as well as possible. The trusted is confronted with a responsibility to handle the dependency of the truster with care. The trusted must use this power in a positive and creative manner, aiming at the well-being of the dependent party, and not abuse the vulnerability that goes with it.[35] The moral moment in the building of trust inheres in the adages "to be trustworthy" and "to put trust in others." The building of trust is thus based on a notion of active responsibility and on the availability of resources to take care of the entrusted goods. Relationality is therefore not only an empirical premise, but also a crucial moral concept in the ethic of care.

Rewriting Familiar Normative Concepts

As we have seen, *independence* is the overarching value in proposed Dutch government policies, just as notions of economic self-sufficiency remain central to Anglo-American debates over reforming welfare states. As Sylvia Bashevkin points out in the introduction to this volume, some feminist arguments for economic independence reflect these same notions of abstract individualism that dominate the distributive paradigm. By way of contrast, my approach presses us to rethink autonomy in a manner that retains the value of economic independence, while simultaneously embedding it in a relational account of human life that deals with actual practices of care and responsibility.

Here the notion of relational autonomy is relevant, since it is based on a descriptive account of "relational selves."[36] People are not viewed as isolated units who live their lives and form their identities apart from others. Instead, individuals need each other in order to live good lives, and can exist as individuals only by engaging in caring relations with others. Individuals develop a "sense of self" because other individuals recognize them and confirm them in their feeling of individuality, value their presence in the world, and make concrete efforts to allow their capabilities to flourish. Selves are not static entities, but are always in process; images of self and other are constantly negotiated and renegotiated in relational contexts. The capacity for autonomy is acquired in contexts where we are dependent on others, can share ideas and beliefs in conversation with others, and can engage in communication in which our experiences and narratives about each other matter. Individual autonomy is, in this respect, a debt to others.[37]

It is useful to distinguish between several subconcepts of autonomy—notably, self-realization and self-determination. Self-realization refers to the ability to develop one's capacities and is connected to the notion of human flourishing. Self-determination, on the other hand, refers to the possibility of making important life decisions without the overt intrusion of others. Self-realization is in many respects intertwined with care, both in terms of care by others and care for the self. We need, therefore, to avoid equating independence with self-sufficiency, since care and responsibility then remain invisible.[38] Even "self-sufficient individuals" have to take account of their responsibilities for others and the care this entails on a daily basis in many situations in their lives.

These remarks have consequences for the notion of independence as employed in debates about work and care. If we see independence as a complex task with which people are faced, instead of as an abstract norm, we could describe it as the capacity to find a balance between care for the self, care for others, and care for the world. Individuals have to find this balance in networks of mutual dependence and responsibility, at home, at work, and in other social contexts. They have to face different forms of dependency and find ways of dealing with them. My own contribution to the discussion of the 1999 white paper "Towards a New Balance between Work and Care" proposed the following reformulation of the central goal of work/care policies: "the attainment of a situation in which everybody can take care of themselves and others, by practicing in the course of their life those combinations between financial responsibility and the responsibility for daily care that fit their situation and needs, and those of the persons who are dependent upon them."[39]

Another thorny normative concept in the discussion is *equality*. Dutch government documents discuss this concept only very briefly, in the context of considering the relationship between equality of outcome or results and equality of opportunity or starting positions. The official position in the Netherlands adopts the latter view, since it accords better with an emphasis on social diversity. This step is remarkable, since the original meaning of equality in public discourse in the 1980s came closer to equality as sameness (erasing the meaning of sexual difference) and thus to a concept of equality of results. It is true that the results-based approach has been criticized from many perspectives, but it is not clear if that critique necessitates a shift toward equality of opportunity. Both concepts of equality follow from an individualistic discourse, geared toward issues like participation in the labor market, access to collective resources, and access to positions of institutional decision-making. The problem with this discourse is, once again, that care is absent from it or is present only in terms of family roles and responsibilities.

I do not wish to imply that the politics of work and care should be stripped of equality norms. On the contrary, a democratic politics of care implies that individuals have equal possibilities in their lives to give and receive care, if we at least accept care as an important social activity. In public debates on health care, I have proposed that access to the public sphere is important, since it is where the politics of needs interpretation takes place and where social arrangements around care can be scrutinized against public standards of accessibility, expediency, and quality of life.[40] Access to care as a relational practice is also significant, since it is here that the values of care are most directly experienced. It would violate social justice norms if specific (including gendered) social groups were privileged in one of these respects. We therefore need a norm of equal opportunities, so that giving and receiving care can be justified with the idea that the possibility of having intimate relations of one's choice is one of the basic values of human life and a crucial condition for human flourishing.

Yet these norms would be meaningless if governments that acknowledged them failed to guarantee a reasonable degree of equality of outcome, as long as the latter were elaborated in a historicized and context-sensitive manner and differentiated for various social groups. It would then be possible to discuss what measures of inequality could prove acceptable, where unequal treatment might be justified, and what trajectory would enhance social equality. Conceptualized in this way, no equality norm necessarily works against diversity. On the contrary, equality norms can accommodate cultural diversity in caring practices and diversity in caring needs very well. In addition, they can challenge structural patterns of privilege and dominance in caregiving and care-receiving, along the lines of gender, class, race, age, and physical condition.

The notion of *freedom of choice* has been used since the 1980s by the Dutch government to justify not adopting "strong measures" in the private lives of citizens. Freedom of choice has been linked to the concept of autonomy, conceived as negative liberty, as a concession not only to free market advocates (who did not welcome redistributive government interventions in labor relations), but also to gay and lesbian movements (that argued for public recognition of alternative lifestyles alongside traditional marriage). Choice thus became a recurring theme of policy documents and began to function as a sort of unreflective shorthand.

What is the meaning of choice from the perspective of care? Policy makers usually work with a conceptual scheme in which ascribed responsibility follows choice. The Dutch government thus assumes that choices for taking on caring responsibilities are "private choices" that ought to be respected. Narratives on care reveal, however, that the "choice" to care is never straightforward. It involves complex dilemmas that may shift and change over time. Future mothers cannot determine in advance the conditions under which they will take care of their children. The health of the children involved cannot be predicted. This uncertainty extends throughout the life cycle. The decision to take care of elderly relatives is in many cases shaped by the relationship with the person in question and by the availability of support from others in the family and community. In most cases, there is not one moment of "choice"; rather, caring is embedded in relationships of increasing dependency and gradual acceptance of it.[41] Caring patterns are often shaped not so much by duty or obligation, but by a sense of commitment that caring is "the proper thing to do."[42]

A democratic ethic of care would argue that people should be able to choose caring arrangements that suit them, that match their needs and values about good care provision. Often, this is not a simple matter. Different parties in the caring process often have conflicting views, and power differences may produce complex forms of dependency. Unwanted forms of dependency between the generations persist when public forms of care for the elderly are not available. In the Netherlands, introducing a carers leave program, important as it may be, does not imply that the problem of care for the frail and elderly is automatically solved.[43] Many elderly people do not want to be dependent on their children or other relatives. The right to choose, in other words, should apply on both sides of the caring relationship.

Choice may also be an empty concept in caring situations in which those who need care are no longer competent to reach well-considered decisions. Even more than in other caring relations, respect for autonomy implies that time, attentiveness, and communicative skills are needed to understand the needs of people dependent on care, as is the case, for example, in caring for Alzheimer patients or severely disabled children. On the whole, what "freedom of choice" regarding care implies, and what it demands from caregivers and care-receivers, should be decided on an individual basis. Politically, this means responsiveness on the part of decision makers to see what is adequate and justifiable. But it also implies that government should ensure that enough realistic possibilities for choice are made available.

These issues all touch on the *relationship between public and private*. It has long been assumed that caring was essentially women's work and women's responsibility, either in the home or in semipublic institutions. A new politics of care, we may conclude from the previous, is a collective responsibility, the basic principle being the social importance of care. This does not imply a complete collectivization of care, however. The Dutch choice under the combination scenario not to opt for a completely collective model is wise, I think, and could form the basis for a new welfare state regime. In this new model, the goal would be to find ways in which different social parties in the care process together stand for good care provision. New collective provisions would be designed that partly socialize care and, at the same time, acknowledge its intimate and relational aspects. After all, daily care has a lot to do with who one is and can be, and thus with issues of identity. It is inherently connected with embodiment and intimacy. It is a dimension of primary relations and the emotional dynamics inherent in them. New policies should also draw new boundaries between the public and the private. After all, the classical meaning of the concept of private is, perhaps for good reason, that of a sphere where one can withdraw from public interference.

This approach implies, finally, that the formal *rights and obligations* that spring from caring relations should be reconsidered. It is not just a principle of equal rights that must set the tone here. If caring is considered as an important social activity, then it justifies a collective responsibility to enable people to engage in caring practices, without being disadvantaged in other respects. This refers to the availability of time, money, and spatial arrangements and to the possibility of developing one's caring capabilities.[44] The integration of "task combining" (as it is called in current Dutch political jargon) in social security law and labor law should be high on the political agenda. There should be, for example, collective provisions against the loss of income and the forgoing of career mobility due to caring responsibilities. This implies the need for a paid carers leave scheme in an integrated notion of social rights.

Together, these remarks point to the need for further developing the notion of care *as a democratic practice* and as a notion of citizenship. We aim to reach beyond the idea of citizenship as a set of rights and duties, in an attempt to find ways of combining the ethic of care with notions of democratic agency.[45] As Joan Tronto has remarked, both caring as intimate involvement with others and caring in broader and more abstract long-term ways are essential to our roles as citizens. Caring requires an involvement both in the intimate relations of daily life and in the more distant relations of public life.[46] In this respect, the demand for equal access to different spheres of life springs from the democratic moral impulse that individuals should have the ability to circulate in different roles and positions, where they can become acquainted with the needs and moral viewpoints of different social actors. If the care ethic is conceived as a political ethic, it would fit into a new social policy paradigm, the contours of which are currently becoming visible at several social sites. This paradigm is a combination of several elements: a coordinating, supportive social state that sets democratic norms and conditions for caring practices; a flourishing civil society in which social movements and semipublic institutions organize a new social infrastructure of care; and a creative space for active forms of citizenship, in which individuals can engage in diverse forms of social commitment that respect human plurality. This is, in fact, the promise that a democratic ethic of care can bring to public life.

Notes

This article was originally presented as a paper at the International Political Science Association conference in Quebec City, in August 2000. I am grateful to Margreth Hoek, Joyce Outshoorn, Jacques Siegers, and Joan Tronto for their encouragement and critical comments. The ideas presented here constitute part of a larger project to reappraise care, sponsored by the Dutch government and based at the University of Utrecht in cooperation with the Dutch Association of Women's Studies. Elements of this paper can be found in several of my Dutch-language publications on the topic, including S. L. Sevenhuijsen, "Naar een nieuwe definitie van zorg," in *Wie zorgt in de 21e eeuw? Jaarboek emancipatie '99*, ed. M. v. S. Zaken (The Hague: Elsevier, 1999); S. L. Sevenhuijsen, "Het combinatiescenario: kansen en bedreigingen voor de toekomst," *Nemesis* 5 (1999): 166–70; and S. L. Sevenhuijsen, "De plaats van zorg. Over de relevantie van zorgehiek voor sociaal beleid" (Utrecht: Utrecht University, 2000).

1. I have applied this method of normative text analysis in S. L. Sevenhuijsen, *Citizenship and the Ethics of Care. Feminist Considerations on Justice, Morality, and Politics* (London: Routledge, 1998), chap. 5; and in S. L. Sevenhuijsen, "Caring in the Third Way: The Relationship between Obligation, Responsibility and Care in Third Way Discourse," *Critical Social Policy* 20 (2000): 5–37.
2. See "Handelingen Tweede Kamer," zitting 1984–1985, 1–2 (The Hague: Beleidsplan Emancipatie, 1985).
3. Ibid., 13.
4. Ibid., 12.
5. See Ministerie van Sociale Zaken em Werkgelegenheid, "Onbetaalde zorg gelijk verdeeld: Toekomstscenario's voor herverdeling van onbetaalde zorgarbeid" (The Hague: Ministerie van Sociale Zaken em Werkgelegenheid, 1995), 79.
6. Ibid., 10, 124.
7. See ibid., 99–127.
8. See Iris Marion Young, *Justice and the Politics of Difference* (Princeton: Princeton University Press, 1990); and Sevenhuijsen, *Citizenship and the Ethics of Care*.
9. Ministerie van Sociale Zaken em Werkgelegenheid, "Onbetaalde zorg gelijk verdeeld," 38.

10. Ibid., 124.
11. Emancipatieraad, "Met zorg naar nieuwe zekerheid" (The Hague: Emancipatieraad, 1996), 26.
12. Ibid.
13. "Handelingen Tweede Kamer," jaar 1996–1997, 25 006, no. 1 (The Hague: Beleidsbrief Emancipatiebeleid, 1997), 13.
14. Ibid., 13–14.
15. Ibid., 14.
16. Ibid., 14.
17. Ministerie van Sociale Zaken en Werkgelegenheid, "Op weg naar een nieuw evenwicht tussen arbeid en zorg" (The Hague: Ministerie van Sociale Zaken en Werkgelegenheid, 1999), 3.
18. See I. Van Staveren, *Caring for Economics: An Aristotelian Perspective* (Delft: Eburon, 1999).
19. See S. Ruddick, *Maternal Thinking: Toward a Politics of Peace* (Boston: Beacon Press, 1989); Joan C. Tronto, *Moral Boundaries: A Political Argument for an Ethic of Care* (New York: Routledge, 1993); and Sevenhuijsen, *Citizenship and the Ethics of Care*.
20. Tronto, *Moral Boundaries*, 103; emphasis in original.
21. See S. L. Sevenhuijsen, "Too Good to Be True? Feminist Considerations about Trust and Social Cohesion," *Focaal* 34 (1999): 207–22; E. F. Kittay, *Love's Labor: Essays on Women, Equality, and Dependency* (New York: Routledge, 1999); and Sevenhuijsen, "De plaats van zorg."
22. Tronto, *Moral Boundaries*, 105.
23. M. Morée, "Wie zorgt straks voor ouderen, zieken en gehandicapten?" In *Wie zorgt in de 21e eeuw?*, ed. v. S. Zaken, 56.
24. In this respect, a democratic ethic of care resembles the human capabilities approach, as elaborated in Martha C. Nussbaum, *Women and Human Development: The Capabilities Approach* (Cambridge: Cambridge University Press, 2000).
25. See Tronto, *Moral Boundaries*, 127.
26. See S. Bickford, *The Dissonance of Democracy: Listening, Conflict, and Citizenship* (Ithaca, N.Y.: Cornell University Press, 1996).
27. Tronto, *Moral Boundaries*, 127.
28. Margaret Urban Walker, *Moral Understandings: A Feminist Study in Ethics* (New York: Routledge, 1998), 107.
29. Ibid., chap. 3.
30. See Sevenhuijsen, *Citizenship and the Ethics of Care*; and Sevenhuijsen, "De plaats van zorg."
31. Tronto, *Moral Boundaries*, 134.
32. Willem Witteveen, *De denkbeeldige staat: Voorstellingen van democratische vernieuwing* (Amsterdam: Amsterdam University Press, 2000), 265.
33. Anette C. Baier, *Moral Prejudices: Essays on Ethics* (Cambridge: Harvard University Press, 1994), 105.
34. Ibid.

35. On the relationship between care and trust, see Sevenhuijsen, "Too Good to Be True;" and Sevenhuijsen, "De plaats van zorg."
36. See C. Mackenzie and N. Stoljar, "Autonomy Refigured," in *Relational Autonomy: Feminist Perspectives on Autonomy, Agency, and the Social Self*, ed. C. Mackenzie and N. Stoljar (New York: Oxford University Press, 2000), 3–31.
37. See L. Barclay, "Autonomy and the Social Self," in *Relational Autonomy*, ed. Mackenzie and Stoljar, 52–71.
38. See Iris Marion Young, *Intersecting Voices: Dilemmas of Gender, Political Philosophy, and Policy* (Princeton: Princeton University Press, 1997), 26.
39. S. L. Sevenhuijsen, "Het combinatiescenario: kansen en bedreigingen voor de toekomst," *Nemesis* 5 (1999): 166–70.
40. See Sevenhuijsen, *Citizenship and the Ethics of Care*, 142–44.
41. E. A. Watson and J. Mears, *Women, Work, and Care for the Elderly* (Aldershot: Ashgate, 1999).
42. J. Finch and J. Mason, *Negotiating Family Responsibilities* (London: Tavistock, 1993).
43. On the details of the elderly care allowance system in the Netherlands as compared with elsewhere in Western Europe, see Jane Jenson's discussion in chapter 3 of this volume.
44. T. Knijn and M. Kremer, "Gender and the Caring Dimensions of Welfare States: Towards Inclusive Citizenship," *Social Politics* 4 (1997): 328–61.
45. See Sevenhuijsen, *Citizenship and the Ethics of Care*; and Joan C. Tronto, *Democratic Caring, Caring for Democracy: Justice, Power, and Inclusiveness*, unpublished manuscript, 1996.
46. Tronto, *Democratic Caring*.

Part II

Confronting Women's Diversity

2.
It's No Longer Just about Race
Social Constructions of American Citizenship in the Moynihan Report

Dionne Bensonsmith

Introduction

The will of the people, or the State, is revealed by the State's institutions. There was not, then, nor is there, now, a single American institution which is not a racist institution. Yes: we have lived through avalanches of tokens and concessions but white power remains white. And what it appears to surrender with one hand it obsessively clutches with the other. I know this is considered heresy.... It translates as meaning that those people who have opted for being white congratulate themselves on their generous ability to return to the slave that freedom which they never had any right to endanger, much less take away.[1]

James Baldwin's 1985 statement from "The Price of the Ticket" reveals much about the role of institutions in structuring citizenship in the United States. Although his writings have largely been ignored by contemporary scholars of American citizenship, essays like "The Price of the Ticket" express the anger and outrage felt by African Americans toward the dismantling of many progressive Great Society programs dating from the 1960s. "The Price of the Ticket" also offers important insights into the influence of race on political institutions and the structure of citizenship. Yet Baldwin's major point that "the will of the people, or the State, is revealed by the State's institutions" begs the crucial question, What do our public institutions reveal about the will of the people and the state with respect to race and gender?

The purpose of this chapter is to discuss broadly the role of one particular American institution, welfare, in structuring beliefs regarding the role of race, sex, and the family in shaping public policy and citizenship. The specific focus is the construction of sex roles and gender in the March 1965 document titled *The Negro Family: The Case for National Action*, commonly known as the Moynihan Report. The report was the work of President Lyndon Johnson's assistant secretary of labor, Daniel Patrick Moynihan, who went on to serve as a prominent Democratic senator from the state of New York. In the report's discussion of black poverty, which Moynihan attributed to the "breakdown of the Negro family," the document constructed African-American women as emasculating matriarchs and reduced sex roles within the family to simplistic binaries between breadwinner/provider (consisting of men) and nurturer/dependents (mainly women).

It is my contention that the Moynihan Report and the debate that ensued over its depiction of the causes and consequences of African-American poverty reveal much regarding contemporary stereotypes of African-American men and women and the relationship between current and past beliefs regarding sex roles and the family. This context helps us to understand better the ways in which social constructions not only affect the debates of which they are a part, but become institutionalized so that they shape future debates as well. Finally, analyzing the Moynihan Report and the controversy that followed its publication helps demonstrate the ways in which social constructions and stereotypes contribute to our beliefs about rights and the obligations of citizenship in the United States.

In addition to reviewing the Moynihan Report, this chapter examines the consequence of the constructions formed in the report for discourses on race, gender, and class. The purpose of this piece is not to assign causality; I am not saying that the Moynihan Report was the sole cause or only source of negative constructions of African-American women and families. Rather, the report drew upon existing racial, sexual, and class stereotypes, highlighting some, such as the idea that African-American women are uncontrollable breeders who cause dysfunction within their families, and submerging others—for example, the long-standing stereotype of the "innocent" but deserted woman who deserves public assistance to help her family. Thus this discussion is also an attempt to place the Moynihan Report, and the constructions contained within it, in historical context. One of the points of this chapter and the larger project of which it is a part is to examine the ways in which the discourse and rhetoric surrounding policy debates like the ones that have occurred over welfare policy contribute to and help structure beliefs regarding race, gender, and citizenship.

The first half of this piece focuses on Moynihan's construction of African-American women and sex/gender roles in the African-American family. For Moynihan, the primary cause of African-American disenfranchisement and the perceived deterioration of the African-American family and, by extension, the black community was the inversion of traditional gender and sex relations between black men and women. As we will see, the Moynihan Report used and expanded stereotypes of African Americans that emerged during slavery, stereotypes that in turn played an influential role in more recent debates during the late 1990s over race, gender, and social policy.

The second half of the analysis considers some possible consequences of the report for discussions of race, gender, and class in America. For example, many of the arguments marshaled in support of reforming welfare in the 1990s reflected the Moynihan Report's traditional constructions of women and proper sex/gender roles within the family. Specifically, the theory that single mother heads of household bred cultural degenerates, social deviants, and pathological behaviors was carefully laid out in the 1965 report. More than just addressing race, then, some of the most negative stereotypes contained in the Moynihan Report were sexist and focused in particular on African-American women. Even though some critics at the time lambasted Moynihan for his depiction of the African-American family and African Americans in general, few devoted sustained attention to his treatment and construction of African-American women and the possible consequences of his construction for gender stereotypes.

A historical examination of the relationship between the constructions contained within the report and other debates over welfare policy reveal the ways in which racial and sexual stereotypes work on a continuum and how varied constructions are ascendant in different historical periods. For instance, in early-twentieth-century debates over mothers' pensions, the predominant stereotype of the target population was that of the "innocent" white widow. This older debate foreshadowed contemporary conflicts between the ideals of the deserving versus undeserving poor. The behavioral characteristics of each group were clear: the category known as deserving poor contained those families that worked for pay but could not get ahead, while the undeserving poor consisted mainly of single mothers of color who bore children out of wedlock. Although these stereotypes remain consistent with contemporary debates, the racial/physical characteristics are distinctly different because race then, unlike now, was defined by ethnicity rather than by genetic phenotype.[2] Many of the changes in the debate over welfare and social policy, specifically those concerning who should receive what types of aid, occurred during the 1960s in the midst of debates over expanding the civil, political, and social rights of African Americans.

Constructing African-American Women: Matriarchy, Independent Women, and the "Tangle of Pathologies"

In the period between the transformation of the Aid to Dependent Children program (established in 1935) into Aid to Families with Dependent Children (AFDC) in 1950 and AFDC's metamorphosis into Temporary Assistance for Needy Families (TANF) in 1996, the discourse on poverty in the United States became increasingly racialized and feminized. In the American welfare state, race is feminized and gender racialized, so that race and gender intersect, meet, and become personified in the images and constructions we have of black women. One of the key documents in this transformation is the Moynihan Report. Published in 1965, at the height of the national debate over the expansion of civil, political, and social rights for African Americans, many of the stereotypes constructed and reconstructed in the report became an integral part of the national lexicon on race and gender in the United States.

Although Daniel Patrick Moynihan wrote *The Negro Family: The Case for National Action* with the stated intent of supporting programs designed to advance rights for African Americans, an *unintended* consequence of his report was the construction of three pernicious stereotypes that would plague African Americans and social policy in later years. These were the emasculating black matriarch, the overly fertile and lazy welfare queen, and the shiftless black male, stereotypes that upon closer inspection have their origins in constructions of African Americans that emerged during slavery. Formed in large part because of the material conditions in which African Americans found themselves while enslaved and as a result of discriminatory laws in the post–Civil War era, these stereotypes later became the "standard" by which conservatives argued for dismantling the same social policies that had been designed to enable African-American enfranchisement.[3]

The following section examines how the Moynihan Report constructed and supported its thesis with respect to sex and gender roles in the family, as well as to matriarchy, black women, and single motherhood. As he developed his thesis regarding the dissolution of the African-American family, Moynihan constructed an argument calling for the "policy of the United States [to] bring the Negro American full and equal sharing in the responsibilities and rewards of citizenship."[4] However, it is through this discussion that the Moynihan Report constructed stereotypes that focused debates over race, gender, and social policy on the dysfunction of female-headed households, rather than on the social, political, and economic structures that were responsible for African-American poverty and disenfranchisement in the first place.

The Influence of Sex and Gender Roles on Family Structure

> There is no one Negro problem. There is no one solution. Nonetheless, at the center of the tangle of pathology is the weakness of the family structure. Once or twice removed, it will be found to be the principal source of most of the aberrant, inadequate, or antisocial behavior that did not establish, but now serves to perpetuate the cycle of poverty and deprivation.[5]

Moynihan began the report by highlighting the perceived disintegration of the black family. He asserted that "the family is the basic social unit of American life; it is the basic socializing unit. By and large, adult conduct in society is learned as a child."⁶ Moynihan thus attempted to explain African-American disenfranchisement by focusing on black behavior and, more specifically, on the structure of African-American families.

He developed this thesis in the following terms:

> The fundamental problem, in which this is most clearly the case, is that of family structure. The evidence—not final, but powerfully persuasive—is that the Negro family in the urban ghettos is crumbling... at the heart of the deterioration of the fabric of Negro society is the deterioration of the Negro family. It is the fundamental source of weakness of the Negro community at the present time.⁷

Moynihan's discussion of sex and gender roles and their effect on family structure posed two arguments. First, it juxtaposed African-American family "types" with those of whites and implied that the behavior of African Americans, especially when it pertained to gender and sex roles in the family, was responsible for black poverty and discrimination. Moynihan did this by setting up binaries between black and white, urban and rural, maleness and femaleness, the "natural" and the "unnatural." In constructing his analysis around binary thinking, the Moynihan Report replicated the "us versus them" dichotomy that has been criticized by scholars of race and gender theory because it consigns blacks—more specifically, black families headed by women—to a lower-class status. Moynihan stated:

> But there is one truly great discontinuity in family structure in the United States at the present time: that between the white world in general and that of the Negro American... The white family has achieved a high degree of stability and is maintaining that stability.⁸

He continued, in bold print, **"by contrast, the family structure of lower class Negroes is highly unstable, and in many urban centers is approaching complete break-down."**⁹ In this way Moynihan also defined what he believed to be the first characteristic of the black lower class, an urban geographical setting.

Juxtaposing white and black children, Moynihan extended the benefit of the doubt to lower-class whites in stating, "white children without fathers at least perceive all about them the pattern of men working. Negro children without fathers *flounder* and *fail*."[10] Furthermore, this statement serves as an example of Moynihan's thinking regarding gender and the family. If we take this statement at face value, the presence of fathers in the home was the most important factor in determining poverty and social dysfunction in families. The presence of a dominant male in the home was followed only by race in the hierarchy of variables that determined economic and social dysfunction within the black community.

Matriarchy: Black Women, Female Heads of Household, and Single-Mother Families

Second, according to Moynihan, African-American disenfranchisement and poverty were attributable to female-headed, so-called broken homes. He cited a litany of statistics in pointing to the rise in separation and divorce rates among "nonwhite" families.[11] These included the following: "nearly a quarter of Negro women living in cities who have ever married are divorced, separated, or are living apart from their husbands ... 26 percent of Negro women ever married are either divorced, separated, or have their husbands absent."[12] Moynihan continued:

> In essence, the Negro community has been forced into a matriarchical structure which, because it is so out of line with the rest of American society, seriously retards the progress of the group as a whole, and imposes a crushing burden on the Negro male and, in consequence, on a great many Negro women as well. There is, presumably, no special reason why a society in which males are dominant in family relationships is to be preferred to a matriarchal arrangement. However, it is clearly a disadvantage for a minority group to be operating on one principle, while the great majority of the population, and the one with the most advantages to begin with, is operating on another.[13]

This statement proposes that more than simply the absence of fathers in the home caused family dysfunction. According to

Moynihan, it was instead the condition of having homes headed by women that contributed to dysfunction and poverty within the black community. For him, the "problem" of female-headed households was so severe that it warranted its own separate section of the report. Moynihan opened his analysis of the "real" cause of problems within the black community with a section that began "Almost one-fourth of Negro families are headed by females."[14]

It must be noted that neither the Moynihan Report nor contemporary discourse on the deviancy/pathology of "broken homes" comments on the status of single-parent families headed by men. We are left to assume either that male-headed single-parent families do not occur, or else that they are free of the dysfunction and pathology associated with lone-parent families headed by women. That dysfunction occurs when women are family heads, regardless of whether a male is present, reveals the double standard applied to men and women with respect to gender and sex roles within the family. Historically, in the discourse on the family, welfare, and social policy, women were considered to be the "harbingers of democracy," the group responsible for socializing little girls and boys into their "proper" gender roles.[15] The primary job of men, then, was to provide the proper financial security so that wives could perform their intended role of taking care of the home, raising the children, and serving husbands.

According to Moynihan, the primary dysfunction in African-American families followed from the fact that the majority of them failed to fit this pattern. He wrote, "a fundamental fact of Negro American family life is the often reversed roles of husband and wife."[16] According to his report, the inversion of gender roles within the African-American family has limited the ability of African Americans to assimilate into the mainstream of American society. Moynihan noted several of these in the report, including the role of slavery and discriminatory post–Civil War legislation (known as Jim Crow laws) in shaping gender roles in the black family. As Moynihan argued, "unquestionably these events worked against the emergence of a strong father figure. The very essence of the male animal, from the bantam rooster to the four-star general, is to strut."[17]

Pointing out the ways in which female heads of household

produce "bad" children, Moynihan observed, "researchers who have focused upon the 'good' boy in high delinquency neighborhoods noted that they typically come from exceptionally stable, intact families." The text continued,

> Recent psychological research demonstrates the personality effects of being reared in a disorganized home without a father. One study showed that children from fatherless homes seek immediate gratification of their desires far more than children with fathers present. Others revealed that children who hunger for immediate gratification are more prone to delinquency, along with less social behavior.[18]

More important for Moynihan, however, was the view that African-American men were *feminized* because of their inability to take their rightful place at the head of the family. To illustrate this point, he cited sociologist Edward Bakke's study of the effects of unemployment on families.

Bakke maintained that the effects of unemployment on family structure could be observed in four stages, "the first two stages end with the exhaustion of credit and the entry of the wife into the labor force. The father is no longer the provider and the elder children become resentful."[19] The third stage was "most critical" for Moynihan, for it was in this period that there "commences a new day-to-day existence." Again quoting Bakke, Moynihan observed:

> At this point two women are in charge: Consider the fact that relief investigators or case workers are normally women and deal with the housewife. Already suffering a loss in prestige and authority in the family because of his failure to be the chief bread winner, the male head of the family feels deeply, this obvious transfer of planning for the family's well-being to two women, one of them an outsider. His role is reduced to that of errand boy to and from the relief office.[20]

To counter the disastrous effects of female-headed households, notably "reduced intelligence, illegitimacy, crime, and delinquency," Moynihan advocated such traditionally masculinizing activities as military service.[21] In addition to providing a place where black men could excel, due to its imposed "meritocracy," Moynihan endorsed military service for black men because "it is an utterly masculine world."[22] He argued:

> Given the strains of the disorganized and matrifocal family life in which so many Negro youth come of age, the Armed Forces are a dramatic and desperately needed change: a world *away from women*, a world run by *strong men* of unquestioned authority; where discipline, if harsh, is nonetheless orderly and predictable, and where rewards, if limited, are granted on the basis of performance.[23]

Moynihan's belief that dependency feminized men had deep historical roots and was consistent with earlier constructions of gender roles that provided the impetus for welfare programs beginning in the late 1800s. In her analysis of the early U.S. welfare state, Gwendolyn Mink (author of chapter 6 in this volume) noted the ways in which welfare proposals and arguments for state-administered social policy often revolved around the perceived relationship between men and women, the masculine and the feminine, and the provider and dependent. Although Mink's analysis considers welfare policy from the late 1800s through the early twentieth century, her observations regarding the construction of the masculine and feminine in welfare policy remain relevant to the Moynihan Report as well. According to Mink,

> By assigning feminine traits to ethnic men, old-stock Americans not only neutered allegedly servile and dependent men but marked them as a peril to republican liberty as well. For while woman's dependency was the mainspring of woman's virtue, men's dependency was the sign of men's inadequacy. The flip side of dependent womanhood was virtuous motherhood; the flip side of dependent manhood was the germ of tyranny.[24]

It is this lack of familial instruction regarding proper sex roles—caused by female dominance in the family and the feminization of black men—that Moynihan identified as the primary cause of political, economic, and social alienation within the African-

American community. It also formed the basis of his call for "a national effort.... that will give a unity of purpose to the many activities of the Federal government in this area, directed to a new kind of national goal: *the establishment of a stable Negro family structure.*"[25]

Criticisms and Defenses of the Moynihan Thesis

Most of the debate that followed the publication of the 1965 report was directed at Moynihan's depiction of the African-American family and his analysis of the causes and consequences of African-American poverty. Very few reviewers took issue with Moynihan's construction of African-American women as emasculating matriarchs or with his ascribed remedies to the "problem" of gender inversion within the African-American family. Early on, critics took note of the potentially negative effects of the report on debates over the causes of and remedies for disenfranchisement within the African-American community. Christopher Jencks summarized many of these critiques in a piece for the *New York Review of Books*:

> Moynihan's analysis is the conservative tradition that guided the drafting of the poverty program.... The guiding assumption is that social pathology is caused less by basic defects in the social system than by defects in particular individuals and groups which prevent their adjusting to the system. The prescription is therefore to change the deviance, not the system.[26]

However, few scholars, journalists, or politicians took issue with Moynihan's depiction of gender/sex roles in the family or with his portrayal of African-American women and the ostensibly deviant households they headed. Although the report drew protest from various leaders, ranging from George Wiley (founder of the National Welfare Rights Organization) to African-American scholars like Robert Staples, most of the critiques focused on Moynihan's analysis of the African-American family. More specifically, critics called into question his depiction of African-American men. The matriarch construction was hotly contested, but this controversy mainly concerned the consequences of such a view for African-American men. Prominent black social scientists, including Joyce Ladner, Andrew Billingsly, Robert Staples, and Angela Davis, refuted Moynihan's depiction of the African-American family as "pathological."[27] Ladner and Billingsly stressed the benefits of a nontraditional family structure, questioning the validity of a white, middle-class family model—given that many of the latter were in crisis due to rebellious and disaffected youth.[28]

As Paula Giddings notes, "though many took issue with Moynihan's view of the problem, however, few criticized his suggestion for resolving it—which was even more malevolent."[29] Specifically, Giddings refers to Moynihan's contention that black men were unsuccessful in the marketplace and with respect to education, while black women, relatively speaking, experienced greater success in both the marketplace and education.

In their book titled *The Moynihan Report and the Politics of Controversy*, Lee Rainwater and William Yancey explained this line of argument as follows: "Moynihan felt that jobs had primacy and that the government should not rest until every able-bodied Negro man was working, even if this meant that some women's jobs had to be redesigned to enable men to fulfill them."[30] Their statement underlines one of the most sexist elements of the report. That is, single-mother heads of households were clearly not the heart of the "Negro problem" for Moynihan; rather, it was the perceived supremacy or parity of black women economically and socially vis-à-vis black men in single-parent *and* dual-parent households that was at issue. Paula Giddings concludes that "the Moynihan Report was not so much racist as it was sexist. Although it can't be held responsible for the intense Black male chauvinism of the period, it certainly didn't discourage it, and the report helped shape Black attitudes."[31]

Giddings, along with a handful of black feminist scholars like Patricia Hill Collins and Wahneema Lubiano, member of the small scholarly community that specifically confronts the sexist constructions contained within the report. It is in the tradition of scholars like Giddings, Hill Collins, and Lubiano that this critique is presented.

Implications for Race, Gender, Public Policy, and Citizenship

Contemporary scholars of race theory have linked the Moynihan Report with the "culture of poverty" thesis espoused by such writers as William Julius Wilson.[32] Notably, Stephen Steinberg, in an article titled "The Liberal Retreat from Race during the Post–Civil Rights Era," chastised William Julius Wilson and his defenders (notably, Michael Katz), calling them an "intellectual reincarnation of Daniel Patrick Moynihan."[33] According to Steinberg,

> In recent years there have been attempts to rehabilitate Moynihan, and to portray him as the hapless victim of the ideological excesses of the sixties.... In point of fact, Wilson struck a number of themes that were at the heart of Moynihan's political analysis in 1965: that blacks had their political rights, thanks to landmark civil rights legislation; that there was "a widening gulf" between the black middle class, which was reaping the benefits of an improved climate of tolerance, and the black lower class, which was as destitute and isolated as ever; that blacks were arriving in the nation's cities at a time when employment opportunities, especially in the manufacturing sector, were declining.... neither Moynihan nor Wilson were advancing a radical theory that challenged structures of inequality, or that envisioned a radical restructuring of major political and economic institutions. All they meant was that lower-class blacks needed to acquire the education and skills that are a prerequisite for mobility and that explain the success of the black middle class.[34]

Steinberg went on to critique what he viewed as the left's capitulation on racial matters to a politics of "everybody." Rather than supporting race-based solutions to race-based problems, Steinberg claimed that one of the more disturbing legacies of the Moynihan Report was the movement away from specific, race-targeted programs for African Americans and toward a focus on personal behaviors as the cause of black disenfranchisement. Observing the disastrous effects of Moynihan's strategy of "semantic infiltration," defined as "the appropriation of the language of one's political opponents and molding it into your own political position for the purposes of blurring distinctions," Steinberg asserted, "only in retrospect can we fully appreciate the dire political implications of suggesting that government programs were futile unless we work to strengthen the family."[35]

Although Steinberg's critiques were on point, they missed the central role that gender constructions played in Moynihan's and Wilson's analyses of black poverty. Both Moynihan and Wilson focused on African-American male employment as one key indicator of well-being in the black family. In so doing, they missed the *gendered* causes of employment discrimination and poverty, which included unequal pay, devaluation of unpaid caring or paid work when viewed as women's responsibilities, the unequal treatment and conditions most women suffered at home and in the workplace, relatively low rates of valuation and pay in professions in which women were well represented (like social work), and female underrepresentation in most of the higher-paying professions and in upper management.[36] The ongoing importance of these factors is revealed throughout this volume, including in Selma Sevenhuijsen's discussion of care policies in chapter 1 and Jane Jenson's analysis of seniors' allowances in chapter 3.

By failing to include gender in his critique, Steinberg missed the opportunity to draw important connections between race, class, and gender that influence the current discourse on poverty policy. For example, Steinberg failed to account for the ways in which gender biases in the study of social policy contributed to the liberal retreat from race. With respect to economic well-being, the fact that leading analysts like Wilson calculate household income based solely on *male* employment obscures the contribution women make to the economic stability of their families. As well, policy debates over affirmative action and reverse discrimination ignore the fact that white women—and, by extension, white families—have benefited directly from affirmative action policies. Including gender in his critique would only have strengthened Steinberg's analysis of the effects of the Moynihan thesis on the liberal retreat from race.

In her article titled "Black Ladies, Welfare Queens, and State Minstrels: Ideological War by Narrative Means," Wahneema Lubiano focused on the gendered legacy of the 1965 report, tracing its effects on subsequent debates involving African-American women. Using as her focal point Anita Hill's testimony before the U.S. Senate Judiciary Committee (when it was considering Clarence Thomas's Supreme Court nomination), Lubiano showed how the matriarch construction employed in the report was used against African-American women. She proposed that Anita Hill's testimony was framed in part within one of the negative stereotypes of African-American women, that of the "black lady." Hill was juxtaposed with Thomas's sister Emma Mae Martin, who as the "welfare queen" represented another long-standing negative stereotype of black women. Important for this analysis, however, is the way in which Lubiano drew parallels between these two stereotypes of black women and their construction in the Moynihan Report.[37] Noting the contributions of the Moynihan Report to both narrative tropes, Lubiano wrote:

> The lesson implied by the Moynihan Report ... in many ways the Ur-text for the simplistic "culture of poverty" discussions as they are represented in the media, is that the welfare-dependent single mother is finally the synecdoche, the shortest possible shorthand, for the pathology of poor, urban, black culture ... the welfare mother is the root of greater black pathology. But the flip side of the pathological welfare queen, as Moynihan's own language tells us, is the other kind of black woman—the black lady, the one whose disproportionate overachievement stands for black cultural strangeness and who ensures the underachievement of "the black male."[38]

Unlike most critics of the Moynihan Report, Lubiano illustrated the complex interplay between race, class, and gender contained within it. She also contributed to the body of knowledge regarding the ways in which social constructions influenced the outcomes of the policy process—in this case, the Senate's confirmation of Clarence Thomas as a Supreme Court justice. More important, Lubiano demonstrated the ways in which dominant stereotypes of African-American women (the welfare queen and the black lady) were bolstered by "official" government documents like the Moynihan Report and worked against black women.

According to Lubiano, when a black woman makes a public claim, as Hill did, we immediately attempt to "categorize" by placing her within the existing paradigm or narrative regarding black women and their societal role. Two of the most identifiable and pernicious stereotypes of black women are those of the welfare queen and the black lady and, as Lubiano demonstrated, both were invoked in the Thomas-Hill fiasco. Of the complex interplay between historical stereotypes of African-American women and the role they play in public discourse, she concluded:

> Across history, and certainly at this moment, one of the most reliable all-purpose scapegoats has been the black woman. In this moment both the "welfare queen" and the "black lady" are pathologies created by an erring state: welfare queens are poor and pathologically dependent because of state-welfare handouts, and black ladies are pathologically independent because state-influenced or assisted affirmative-action programs keep such ladies from what they might otherwise become: the spousal appendages of successful black patriarchs.[39]

While both Steinberg and Lubiano illustrated the political and social consequences of the Moynihan thesis for discourses on race, poverty, and gender, they overlooked the policy and institutional consequences of the document. Its main thrust was aptly summarized in the subtitle *The Case for National Action*, which helped to provide the justification for extending government intervention from the public realm of institutional structures that caused poverty and disenfranchisement to the personal domain of the family and the individual. Moynihan's opening statement bears repeating for, like any introduction, it established the tone and summarized the main idea of the report:

> The fundamental problem, in which this most clearly is the case, is that of family structure. The evidence—not final, but powerfully persuasive—is that the Negro family in the urban ghettos is crumbling.... A national effort is required that will give a unity of purpose to the many activities of the Federal government in this area, directed to a new kind of national goal: the establishment of a stable Negro family structure.[40]

These statements bring to light one possible reason for sustained comparisons between black and white families in the report. That is, the 1965 document prescribed for black families a course of action that remains anathema to core American values, since it entails government intervention in the private sphere of the family. It is important to note that Moynihan justified this action, and built his entire argument, on the backs of the black woman. It was her perceived dominance within the black family that provided the impetus for drastic government action and justified the state's insertion into the role of enforcer, father, assimilator, and authority figure in the black family.

Contemporary Echoes of the Report

My point is not to argue for strict divisions between public and private spheres. Instead, my intent is to illuminate some important inconsistencies within the Moynihan analysis, inconsistencies that are all the more interesting given the recent revival of the Moynihan thesis by conservative scholars and politicians.[41] The fact that conservative politicians like Newt Gingrich, who served after 1994 as Republican speaker of the U.S. House of Representatives, and conservative scholars like Lawrence Mead so rigorously endorsed the violation of one of the basic tenets of liberalism—the right to individual privacy—by itself suggests the Moynihan Report deserves a close second look.

For the purposes of this discussion, I will examine Lawrence Mead's analysis of poverty, race, and citizenship in his book called *Beyond Entitlement*. Mead's ideas figured prominently in the 1996 U.S. welfare reform bill, known as the Personal Responsibility and Work Opportunity Reconciliation Act, which is considered in chapter 5 by Sylvia Bashevkin, chapter 6 by Gwendolyn Mink, and chapter 7 by Leah F. Vosko. Evaluating his work brings into focus some of the more punitive parts of this legislation, including its strict work requirements for single mothers, the time limiting of welfare to only two consecutive years and five years lifetime total, and the expansion of social assistance to two-parent households (the only part of the U.S. social welfare system that was expanded in the 1996 legislation).[42]

Although Mead's stated purpose in *Beyond Entitlement* was to press for a scaling back of the Great Society programs that Moynihan advocated in 1965, a closer examination reveals that while their intentions may have been different, both authors constructed their arguments in similar terms. There exist clear continuities between Mead's 1987 description of the problem of the underclass and the policies he advocated to alleviate them and Moynihan's 1965 depiction of African-American families. Moynihan and Mead are remarkably close on two points. First, both called for government intervention into the private lives of the "underclass" for the purpose of setting rules, giving structure, enforcing "good values," and assimilating the "lesser" classes into the American mainstream. Second, both authors racialized and sexualized the underclass.

Mead depicted the underclass as a group that required the repeal of "liberal" social programs and the imposition of a strict, morally rigid, reductive program of "rules and obligations" to teach mainstream American values.[43] Mead wrote:

> There is substantial agreement about the nature of the social problem. A class of Americans, heavily poor and nonwhite, exists apart from the social mainstream.... The underclass is most visible in urban slum settings and is about 70 percent nonwhite, but includes many rural and white people as well, especially in Appalachia and the South. Much of the urban underclass is made up of street hustlers, welfare families, drug addicts, and former mental patients.[44]

Mead went on to draw stronger connections between the underclass and African Americans, making the connection between his ideas and Moynihan's even tighter. He observed:

> The disadvantaged are seen as people who already function marginally and may become lower-class unless their "deficits" in income and skills are dealt with.... Yet much of the real concern, as with disadvantage, stems from the belief that poverty causes problems such as crime or family breakup that are much more damaging to integration. An even more important group to federal policymakers has been nonwhites, especially blacks, who have been

the "special objects and beneficiaries" of federal policy since the civil rights movement.... policymaking attention has focused mainly on that share of black America with the income and behavioral problems associated with the underclass.... While there is no necessary connection between race and lower-class status, blacks do face special difficulties because so many members of their group have functioning problems.[45]

Although Mead set himself apart from Moynihan as a critic of Lyndon Johnson's Great Society, his analysis rests very much in the same tradition. In a chapter mistitled "Functioning, the New Shape of the Social Problem," Mead, like Moynihan, blamed poverty and social dysfunction on the black matriarch and her male counterpart, the street hustler. Pitting middle-class blacks against lower-class blacks, he stated:

[A] bifurcation has occurred in black America. While better-prepared blacks have made good use of fairer opportunity to get ahead, large numbers have also descended into the underclass. The share of black families headed by women rose from 21 to 41 percent between 1960 and 1982.... [t]he effect of family breakup was to reverse black economic gains, since female headed families are usually thrown onto welfare.... Though the gap between white and black *earnings* is closing, the gap in *family income* between the races is now growing largely because of black female-headedness.[46]

Finally, like his predecessor, Mead advocated government programs that would intervene in the "private" sphere so as to change the behavior of underclass members—assimilating them so that they fell in line with mainstream American values. For Mead, like Moynihan, this process was not just a matter of economic necessity, but also a moral imperative to help invigorate the lesser classes with the codes of behavior more in line with "functioning" American citizens.

"The will of the state," in James Baldwin's terms, is expressed by the government's ability to create and maintain a uniform citizenry.[47] One of the roles of the welfare state, then, is to assimilate those who can blend into the mainstream and contain others who cannot absorb the social, economic, and political behaviors of mainstream American society.[48] This is one way that the welfare state has affected the shape and quality of American citizenship. As Mead concluded,

> In the past the nation transcended its fears of federal authority because common citizenship was ultimately more important than freedom.... That citizenship made limited but definite demands. It respected differences of cultural background but insisted on the competences, such as working and speaking English, that were essential to constitute a single society, at least in political and economic affairs.... Nation-building has in fact been an important goal of social policy. The Great Society policy was an attempt to redefine the terms of belonging in American society to encompass, more surely than before, the poor, the disadvantaged, and the nonwhite.... The difficulty, of course, was that it no longer sufficed to liberate people to achieve this.... The libertarian reflexes of federal politics served the cause of equal citizenship when rights were threatened; they endanger it when the need is for firmer requirements. Somehow the rhetoric of equal rights that dominates federal politics must be turned around to justify equal obligations as well.[49]

That this intervention is prescribed for certain groups and not others, and that groups are defined by their racial and sexual characteristics, is a matter for caution and concern. Although scholars like Mead claimed that enacting stricter social programs would help to equalize our society, they ignored the fact that these claims are justified with racist and sexist stereotypes that hold racist and sexist effects.

Perhaps this was their objective. In the politics of the welfare state, racial and sexual divisions appear not only as common fare, but also as required practice if one is to argue for social policies. The idea that the "dialogue" around social policy has been determined between the boundaries of race, class, and gender has not been lost on social policy theorists. One has only to review studies of the U.S. welfare state and the construction of citizenship to know that gender and race have supplied the crucial subtext in debates over the development of that state.[50] While scholars have performed the much-needed task of explicating the ways in which the welfare state structures citizenship in relation to, and in some cases in opposition to, beliefs about race, they have ignored the one group upon whom the foundation of most U.S. debates about welfare is built—that is, African-American women.

Both Gwendolyn Mink and Suzanne Mettler noted the ways in which the social rights of male citizens have been expanded, in large part by government intervention into the private sphere for the purposes of protecting women.[51] Yet they failed to note the ways in which theorists and architects of the American welfare state have expanded citizenship rights by arguing for government intervention in the "private" sphere in order to rectify dysfunctions in the African-American community. A closer inspection of the *rhetoric* that surrounded changes in social policy in the 1960s reveals that many Great Society programs were enacted to alleviate perceived personal and social dysfunctions in the African-American community, dysfunctions whose primary cause, according to the Moynihan Report, was the inversion of gender and sex roles in the African-American family. Because these scholars only tangentially addressed the specific conditions of African-American women with respect to social policy, they missed one important facet of what Mettler described as the ever-expanding "tent of American citizenship."[52] Specifically, they missed the fact that while the expansion of the tent was often justified in the name of racial and sexual inclusion, the effects have been woefully short in advancing this goal.

Although the expansion of social and political rights that occurred in the 1960s (via affirmative action policies and Title IX of the Civil Rights Act) pulled a significant number of white women—and, by default, white Americans—into the economic and political tent, African Americans and other peoples of color still find themselves left out. Black women remain at the bottom of the heap for "every indicator of social, economic, and political well-being."[53] As this chapter points out, it remains one of the major paradoxes of welfare state development that gains in citizenship rights have been made, in part, on the basis of arguments that are largely racist and sexist. And to further explain one of the more exploitative aspects of American social policy, these gains have used negative stereotypes of African Americans—specifically, parodied constructions of African-American women—to benefit already privileged groups.

Conclusion

Just as the social constructions of African-American women in welfare policy and in the Moynihan Report help us to understand developments in the U.S. welfare state, they also shed light on evolving ideas about race, gender, class, and citizenship. Social constructions in the welfare state act as more than a rhetorical device for politicians, scholars, and reformers. Social constructions can operate as an organizing device through which we decide "who gets what, when, and how."[54] Through our political institutions, social constructions also organize citizenship, parsing out which citizens can make claims on the state and what types of claims are considered legitimate.

The Moynihan Report and subsequent writings about welfare, including Lawrence Mead's *Beyond Entitlement*, explicitly construct welfare recipients in terms of their perceived racial, sexual, and behavioral characteristics. These constructions not only symbolize what James Baldwin called "the will of the people or the State," regarding what we value, the types of behavior we want to encourage, and by whom, but they also are instructive. Social policy conveys meaning to the larger public. Like the maternalist reformers of the 1920s and 1930s, welfare reformers in the 1960s and 1990s helped to advance a cultural and assimilationist concept of race and gender.

In explicating the characteristics that make up the under and lower classes, and by constructing them in *racial* and *sexual* terms, documents like the Moynihan Report helped to define which characteristics and behaviors were, over time, associated with African Americans versus whites. In that 1965 document, race was not simply phenotype, but rather was constructed around and constituted characteristics that were definable by values, actions, and behaviors beyond those of physical appearance.

From the 1960s to the present, race debates and discussions

about welfare have centered around the construction of "American values."⁵⁵ The Moynihan Report helped to define these values. More important, Moynihan's discourse on welfare went even further in articulating and constructing white identity and behavior. Scholars have observed the ways in which African Americans, even upon adopting the desired characteristics of American citizens, still fail to assimilate into the mainstream of American life. In this way, the constructions and stereotypes of African Americans that emerged during debates over welfare went further to help explain, inform, and instruct white identity. Social constructions like that of the welfare queen instructed Americans in general, and white Americans in particular, about the behaviors and characteristics that comprised the "good" versus deficient citizen.

The discourse surrounding the welfare state has thus constructed and offered lessons about gender and race roles. Welfare policy teaches white women the desired heterosexual behaviors by juxtaposing and constructing the deviant black welfare queen, who is sexually and socially independent from men. Moynihan's black matriarch operated as an example to white women of what too much independence brought—namely, poverty, male abandonment, crime, and illegitimacy.[56]

While the particular institutional arrangements created by the 1935 U.S. Social Security Act (which created the Aid to Dependent Families program) played a pivotal role in structuring both welfare policies and citizenship along race and gender lines, subsequent social constructions had an equally important influence. The discourse of the 1965 Moynihan Report regarding welfare, crime, and illegitimacy helped to refine these characteristics with respect to race and gender and continues to influence debates over welfare state arrangements, policy designs, and citizenship in the United States.

Notes

1. James Baldwin, "The Price of the Ticket," in *Baldwin: Collected Essays* (New York: Library of America, 1998), 839.
2. See Gwendolyn Mink, "The Lady and the Tramp: Gender, Race, and the Origins of the American Welfare State," in *Women, the State, and Welfare*, ed. Linda Gordon (Madison: University of Wisconsin Press, 1990), 92–122; and Linda Gordon, *Pitied but Not*

Entitled: Single Mothers and the History of Welfare (New York: Free Press, 1994).

3. In his 1966 reply to Moynihan, Frank Riessman effectively summed up the intent and consequences of the report:

    I am convinced that Daniel Moynihan is sincerely opposed to discrimination and his report is intended to document its negative consequences.... however, the report represents a highly inappropriate approach to the development of programs and policy to fulfill the rights of the Negro." (Frank Riessman, "In Defense of the Negro Family," *Dissent* [March–April 1966]: 266–267.)

4. Office of Policy Planning and Research, United States Department of Labor, *The Negro Family: The Case for National Action* (hereafter referred to as the Moynihan Report; Washington, D.C., March 1965), 48.
5. Ibid., 30.
6. Ibid., 5.
7. Ibid.
8. Ibid.
9. Ibid.
10. Ibid., 35 (emphasis added).
11. Ibid., 8.
12. Ibid., 8.
13. Ibid., 29.
14. Ibid., 9.
15. Gwendolyn Mink, *The Wages of Motherhood: Inequality in the United States, 1917–1942* (Ithaca, N.Y.: Cornell University Press, 1995), 3–27.
16. Moynihan Report, 31.
17. Ibid., 6.
18. Ibid., 39.
19. Ibid.,19.
20. Ibid.
21. Ibid., 39.
22. Ibid., 42.
23. Ibid., 43.
24. Mink, "The Lady and the Tramp," 96.
25. Moynihan Report, preface, n.p.
26. Christopher Jencks's review of the Moynihan Report, initially published in the *New York Review of Books* (October 14, 1965), as quoted in Lee Rainwater and William L. Yancey, eds., *The Moynihan Report and the Politics of Controversy* (Cambridge: MIT Press, 1967), 217.
27. See Paula Giddings, *When and Where I Enter: The Impact of Black Women on Race and Sex in America* (New York: William Morrow, 1984), 328–29.
28. Giddings, *When and Where I Enter*, 326.
29. Ibid., 328.
30. Rainwater and Yancey, *The Moynihan Report and the Politics of Controversy*, 29.

31. Giddings, *When and Where I Enter*, 329.
32. See William Julius Wilson, *The Truly Disadvantaged* (Chicago: University of Chicago Press, 1987).
33. Stephen Steinberg, "The Liberal Retreat from Race during the Post–Civil Rights Era," in *The House That Race Built*, ed. Wahneema Lubiano (New York: Pantheon, 1997), 13–43.
34. Ibid., 31.
35. Ibid., 22.
36. See Margaret Weir, *Politics and Jobs: The Boundaries of Employment Policy in the United States* (Princeton: Princeton University Press, 1992); and Claudia Goldin, *Understanding the Gender Gap: An Economic History of American Women* (New York: Oxford University Press, 1990).
37. Wahneema Lubiano, "Black Ladies, Welfare Queens, and State Minstrels: Ideological War by Narrative Means," in *Racing Justice, Engendering Power*, ed. Toni Morrison (New York: Random House, 1992), 323–63.
38. Ibid., 335.
39. Ibid., 354.
40. Moynihan Report, preface, n.p.
41. See E. J. Dionne, *They Only Look Dead: Why Progressives Will Dominate the Next Political Era* (New York: Touchstone, 1996); and Michael Lind, *Up from Conservatism: Why the Right Is Wrong for America* (New York: Free Press, 1996).
42. Mead testified twice before Congress to advocate more conservative, work-centered welfare reform proposals. For a transcript of his 1995 testimony before the House of Representatives Ways and Means Subcommittee on Human Resources, see *Contract with America—Welfare Reform* (Hearing before the Subcommittee on Human Resources of the Committee on Ways and Means, House of Representatives, 104th Cong., 2 February 1995, Serial 104-43).
43. Lawrence Mead, *Beyond Entitlement: The Social Obligations of Citizenship* (New York: Free Press, 1986).
44. Ibid., 21, 22.
45. Ibid., 23, 24.
46. Ibid., 36.
47. Baldwin, "The Price of the Ticket," 841.
48. For an analysis of this concept, see Frances Fox Piven and Richard Cloward, *Regulating the Poor: The Functions of Public Welfare*, 2nd ed. (New York: Vintage, 1993).
49. Mead, *Beyond Entitlement*, 256–57.
50. See Barbara J. Nelson, "The Origins of the Two-Channel Welfare State: Workmen's Compensation and Mothers' Aid," in *Women, the State, and Welfare*, ed. Gordon, 123–51; Suzanne Mettler, *Dividing Citizens* (Ithaca, N.Y.: Cornell University Press, 1998); Robert C. Lieberman, *Shifting the Color Line: Race and the American Welfare State* (Cambridge: Harvard University Press, 1998); and Jill Quadagno, *The Color of Welfare: How Racism Undermined the War on Poverty* (Oxford: Oxford University Press, 1994).

51. See Mink, "The Lady and the Tramp"; and Mettler, *Dividing Citizens*.
52. Mettler, *Dividing Citizens*, 1–27.
53. See Deborah Gray White, *Ar'n't I a Woman? Female Slaves in the Plantation South* (New York: Norton, 1999), 23.
54. Harold Laswell, *Who Gets What, When, and How?* (New York: McGraw Hill, 1936).
55. See Lind, *Up from Conservatism*; and Dionne, *They Only Look Dead*.
56. Patricia Hill Collins argues that it was no coincidence that the matriarch construction emerged and gained prominence at the same time that the women's movement began to tackle issues of economic and social equality. See Patricia Hill Collins, *Black Feminist Thought: Knowledge, Consciousness, and the Politics of Empowerment* (New York: Routledge, 1991), 79.

3.
Paying for Caring
The Gendering Consequences of European Care Allowances for the Frail Elderly

Jane Jenson

Introduction

In Western Europe, the redesigned welfare states of the 1990s have increasingly recognized age-related dependence as an "average risk." It is therefore being addressed in ways similar to other risks—such as unemployment or illness—against which post-1945 social citizenship already provided some protection. Just as earlier periods of reform generated a variety of patterns and a range of welfare state regimes, so, too, are countries following different paths as they move to address the needs of the frail elderly—most of them women. The consequences for gender relations and gender inequalities are as varied in this realm as they are in more familiar social policy areas such as welfare and child-care policy.

One direction of contemporary reform has been to include *payments for care* for the frail elderly in a basket of publicly financed social and health services. Germany, the Netherlands, and Japan, for example, have introduced universal insurance schemes to cover long-term care, both residential and domiciliary. Austria has a universal system of care allowances, financed out of general revenues. Other countries are simply incorporating home care and care benefits into existing programs, some of which are universal and some of which are more narrowly targeted. Thus, France has added a needs-based program for residential and home care to the menu of options available to the frail elderly, while Finland and the United Kingdom have introduced attendant allowances to their program mix.

This chapter examines the allowances and other forms of payment for care that are being developed in a context of both rising numbers of frail elderly and ongoing pressures to redesign welfare states. Five areas of care and assistance for older people exist in advanced industrial systems: help at home, institutional care, auxiliary care, housing, and support for informal care.[1] When they are paid to cover some of the costs of dependence, elder care allowances enable frail seniors to purchase services or, in some cases, to transfer a sum of money to a caregiver, including people who provide care informally. Some jurisdictions have opted for another form of allowance that is paid directly to the care provider (see table 3.1).

Table 3.1: Payments for Care: Paid to Frail Elderly and/or Caregivers

	Name	Means Tested and Needs Tested?	Paid to the Dependent Person	Unrestricted Use Unrestricted Access	Paid to the Caregiver	Caregiver Gains Access to Social Security and Labor Rights
Germany (insurance)	Pflegegeld Dependency allowance	N	✓	✓+		✓
Austria (insurance)	Pflegegeld Dependency allowance	N	✓	✓		✓
Denmark	Plejevederlag Caregiver allowance	N		✓	✓	✓
Finland	Omaisloidon Allowance to employ a caregiver	N	✓	✓	✓	✓
	Elkensaajien hoiotuki Dependency allowance	N		✓		
France	Prestation spécifique Dépendance Dependency allowance	N and M	✓	✗		✓
Netherlands	Persoonsgebonden budget Allowance to employ a caregiver	N	✓	✗	✓	✓
	Loopbaanonderbreking Family leave	N		✗	✓	✓
United Kingdom	Attendancts' Allowance Allowance to employ a caregiver	N	✓			
	Invalid Care Allowance Caregiver allowance	N and M		✗	✓	✗

Sources: Rostgaard and Fridberg, 1998; Jenson and Jacobzone, 2000.
+The amount of the benefit is higher if the person uses formal services.

In most cases in Western Europe, payments for care—whether paid to the elderly person as an attendant allowance or to the care provider as a care allowance—give carers access to social security systems, if they choose to register. No matter the details of the design, therefore, such programs have prompted a transfer of some care work from the informal to the formal sector, thereby changing the relationship between some women caregivers and the paid labor force and altering relationships within the family economy as well.

The central proposition of this discussion is as follows. By creating elder-care allowances, policy makers are doing more than creating social programs. They are making choices about how to redesign the citizenship regime and are determining the model of gender relations encoded within it. Therefore, this chapter examines the consequences of elite policy choices for gender relations and explores the likely shape of the new citizenship regime that is emerging from these additions to the benefit and service basket of West European welfare states.

Welfare States and Care Work

In recent years, the welfare state has been commonly defined as an institution designed to ensure the decommodification of labor, meaning a set of programs and policies whose goal was to free workers from the discipline of the labor market.[2] This description has historical validity, but it is also the representation of history as written by those who celebrate the successes of social democracy and a triumphant working class. Other ways of reading the same history of the welfare state are possible.[3] A different lens might allow us to see that social movements, including the workers' movement, claimed *access to care* as a right of social citizenship. Indeed, a wide range of social programs addresses the risk of dependency and the need for care. According to this view, unemployment insurance loses its status as the fundamental program of the welfare state, while programs providing public health care and pensions move to the forefront.

We can identify several specific goals of social programs related to care. One is the effort to redistribute the risk of differential needs for care. Family policy that redistributes the financial burden of raising children provides one example, as do insurance schemes or services provided to the frail elderly, which compensate for the costs of dependence. A second set of programs seeks to improve the quality of care, by regulating service providers, for instance, or by professionalizing care. Finally, there exist programs that aim to reduce what is viewed as dependency and sustain what is seen as autonomy. Pensions for the elderly, for example, ostensibly allow individuals to care for themselves and not be dependent on their families. Housing and income support for the elderly fall into this same category.

The programs mentioned here, and many others, have arisen as responses to the "social question" at least since the nineteenth century. They reflect preoccupations with the issue of care in old age, in childhood, and in sickness, as well as concerns over the problem of dependence on charitable or second-class care that can befall people who are poor, disabled, or otherwise in need.

Questions about how to care for the frail elderly were raised in this same context. The usual answer to the question, Who cares? was "the family," especially women within it. As Selma Sevenhuijsen argues in chapter 1, informal care by daughters, wives, and other female relatives has long been—and remains—by far the most prevalent way of providing for the needs of frail elderly persons. Nonetheless, alongside this type of care existed another kind. For most of the postwar period, professional health care in long-term institutions was offered as a social right of citizenship in most West European countries. For the frail elderly, this arrangement meant that care was provided in hospitals or residential institutions *if* families could no longer care for them.

Over time, the issue of publicly financed and, in some cases, publicly provided, home care gradually appeared on the policy agenda. In recent years, sociological changes such as rising rates of female labor force participation and demographic shifts involving an aging population led many welfare states to try to combine institutional with community care, thus creating a mix of public and private responsibility.[4]

In current debates about home care and how to divide the labor involved in elder care between the informal sector (that is, the family) and the formal sector, we see the extent to which access to health care remains a core dimension of European social citizenship, even as it takes on different forms. It is therefore important to explore and assess the consequences for gender relations of this redistribution of responsibility within the welfare triangle of state, market, and family. Given that these are long-standing concerns, they provide an excellent window for reading the ways in which citizenship regimes are being redefined as new patterns of equality and inequality emerge.

Care and Citizenship Regimes

Since at least 1945, welfare states have been concerned with the distribution of responsibility for caring work, the costs of care, and types of services. Since this corresponds with the time when T. H. Marshall first identified the establishment of social rights of citizenship, we are led to examine closely the notion of citizenship and its connection to care and especially caring work. In peering through this window, to make sense of the immensely rich variety of new and old programs, we will use the concept of *citizenship regime*.[5] This notion refers to the institutional arrangements, rules, and understandings that guide concurrent policy decisions and expenditures by states, problem definitions by states and citizens, and claims-making by citizens.[6]

The concept of citizenship regime stands on two theoretical legs. One is the historical-institutionalist approach to comparative politics.[7] Embedded in this approach is an analytic proclivity for uncovering and attributing importance to ideas, as well as to practices.[8] A citizenship regime encodes within it a set of identities, of the "national" or "model citizen," the "second-class citizen," and the noncitizen. It contributes to a definition of politics that organizes the boundaries of political debate and problem recognition in each jurisdiction. It encodes representations of the proper and legitimate social relations among and within categories and establishes the borders of public and "private."

The second theoretical leg of this concept is the regulation school notion of stability and change in the patterning of social relations.[9] Without revisiting this approach to political economy in any detail, suffice it to say that regulationists claim that some historical moments have sufficient stability in basic social, economic, and political relations to allow regimes to reproduce themselves. At other times, crisis provokes profound redirection. Organizing and legitimating principles break down, and alternative institutional arrangements, rules, and understandings are promoted.

Standing on both of these theoretical legs leads us to pay attention to systems of ideas, the institutions in which they are embedded, and the actions of a variety of actors, each with their own interests. In particular, the dimension of time is essential. Where stability and change are the focus, it is absolutely necessary to pay close attention to social and political processes as they unfold through time and as processes of change take hold.

It is also essential that we give some content to the notion of citizenship regimes. Following T. H. Marshall, we can define the central idea of post-1945 citizenship regimes as ensuring that everyone is treated as a full and equal member of society.[10] Marshall's own prescription for achieving equal treatment was the British welfare state. For him,

> by guaranteeing civil, political, and social rights to all, the welfare state ensures that every member of society feels like a full member of society, able to participate in it and enjoy the common life of society. Where any of these rights are withheld or violated, people will be marginalized and unable to participate.[11]

As the myriad studies devoted to issues of citizenship and welfare states demonstrate, there is very little agreement about the kind of rights needed, the forms of political participation and access entailed, or even the feeling of belonging that results from welfare state development.[12] Yet despite the varied results of nationally specific trajectories, equality was in every case a central value, just as the emphasis on social rights was widespread in the welfare states created at the time.

By the late 1990s, the notion that full citizenship required a commitment to equality of social rights became very widely contested. Indeed, we were much more likely to hear that citizenship was about recognition of differences, or simply about equality in civil rights and access to political power, than that it concerned social equality.[13] Such debates and contestation about the future force us to recognize that, as Dionne Bensonsmith argues with reference to the past in chapter 2, citizenship has always been a social construction. Out of political controversy and competition for power come the two major dimensions of any citizenship regime. These are, first, the relationship between the state and the individual citizen, particularly the rights to which citizens are entitled and the role of the state in guaranteeing these rights. The second dimension involves the division of labor among the state, the market, and the family. Indeed, values expressed via this dimension of the citizenship regime identify matters as being rights of citizens, rather than goods or services to be acquired through market behavior or via "private" family relations.

Preferences for an active state, for example, tend to displace market mechanisms for distributing personal services and transform them into a citizens' right to a public service, with distribution decided by mechanisms of democratic control and carried out by civil servants. Indeed, we can define social policy as "the use of political power to supersede, supplement, or modify operations of the economic system in order to achieve results which the economic system would not achieve on its own."[14] By way of contrast, as Maureen Baker demonstrates in chapter 4, ideological enthusiasm for the market will provoke market-mimicking behavior among public authorities and will make citizens' access to services a matter of their own market capacity. In the realm of health care, for example, a statist preference might well lead to a universal system, while a market emphasis would probably generate a mixed system, in which elements of public insurance were combined with private insurance and spending from one's own private resources.

A single phenomenon, observed over time, can be exceedingly instructive for appreciating the relationship between citizenship regimes and the current moment of economic and social turbulence. The focus of this chapter is the change over time in the ways that provision of care for the frail elderly intersects with gender equality, both as discourse and practice.

Economic autonomy, including the right to enter into a labor contract and earn an income by one's labor, is one of the most basic civil rights, long claimed by women's movements and their allies.

Most men gained this right with the final collapse of feudalism and its replacement by a market for labor, in eighteenth- and nineteenth-century Europe. Women, especially married women, gained the same individual right only after World War II. In more recent decades, the distinction between formal and real equality came to the fore in this as in so many other domains of citizenship. Given the complex linkages between caregiving and employment in their lives, women's equality in the labor market is no more than formally achieved until the matter of care work is settled.[15]

The balance of this chapter's discussion examines how care claims have fared, as citizenship regimes have been restructured in the face of the breakdown of the postwar consensus about the respective role of states, markets, and families. It examines in detail the fate of the equality agenda, as well as the relative responsibility of states and markets in the provision of publicly financed and publicly provided care for the dependent elderly versus private familial or commercial provision.

Marketizing Care Allowances for the Dependent Elderly

Despite the attention paid to care in welfare states, particularly during the three decades after 1945, the frail elderly and their long-term care needs were not at the center of thinking about public services and welfare states. Most seniors were cared for "invisibly" by the women of the family. The social rights of citizenship, whether on an insurance or a universal base, rarely included full access to long-term care.[16] Some services were available, but they tended to be provided by charitable or religious bodies or as "last resort" municipal social assistance. Thus, even if such programs had some public financing, they were rarely imbued with the values of social citizenship.[17]

Welfare triangles that placed a heavy emphasis on family provision created what some observers called an "invisible welfare state" of informal care work by women.[18] This unpaid labor provided for the needs of the dependent, whether children or the frail elderly. Rapidly rising rates of female labor force participation since the 1960s did not eliminate this invisible welfare state by any means; in fact, four-fifths of all care provided to the frail elderly in some parts of Western Europe remains informal.[19] Indeed, many care providers are sandwiched between paid work and care work, between caring for children and caring for their frail elderly relatives. They are, as study after study reveals, confronted with a situation in which caring responsibilities compete with their own employment, a rivalry that sometimes leads to their full withdrawal from the labor force and at other times to reduced hours or less demanding jobs. To the extent that trade-offs must be made, both mounting levels of reliance on informal care and the policy choice of assigning more long-term care responsibilities to the family and community constitute a potential menace to women's chances of achieving economic self-sufficiency. Parallel with Selma Sevenhuijsen's argument in chapter 1, these developments suggest that it is impossible to divorce debates about women's labor market experiences and citizenship status from discussions of caregiving and care-receiving.

Of course, even in the postwar years, some care was provided outside the family. At first, it was primarily institutional care, available either to people whose families could not provide for them or to frail seniors without family. Once the interest in "community care" options increased, efforts were made to relocate care for the dependent elderly in the community, providing it as professional home care or in sheltered communities. In the Nordic countries in particular, a shift in provision occurred so that care was delivered by municipalities or other institutions of home help and housing. We see this same legacy in data from the early 1990s that showed a high proportion of home help in the "care mix" for persons over sixty-five years of age in Denmark, Sweden, and Finland. In Germany and France, by way of contrast, children and spouses provided most of the care.[20]

After 1975, policy makers throughout Western Europe had to rethink earlier policy choices. A new interest in "payments for care" was expressed in the 1980s and 1990s. As table 3.2 shows, this shift rarely entailed a commitment to gender equality or a desire to address the inequalities reproduced by an unequal gender division of labor in the family (essentially the feminization of unpaid work, parallel with the feminization of low-paid work in the regular labor market). Rather, decisions to create such benefits were often a

Table 3.2: Announced Objectives of Payments for Care

	Policy objectives
Germany	Keep the frail elderly at home as long as possible; reduce the demand for institutional care Reduce the demand for social assistance Free children and families from family responsibilities Stimulate the development of social networks Recognize informal care as "work"
Austria	Keep the frail elderly at home as long as possible Express solidarity toward those living in a situation of dependency Increase choice about services Encourage the use of informal care
Denmark	Provide a family leave Keep the frail elderly at home as long as possible Increase choice about services Stimulate the development of social networks
Finland	Keep the frail elderly at home as long as possible *Omaisloidon*—Provide some remuneration to the caregiver for the loss of income *Elkensaajien hoiotuki*—Provide some remuneration of the extra costs of dependency
France	Keep the frail elderly at home or help them to cover the costs of institutional care Create jobs; reduce unemployment
Netherlands	Provide a family leave *Persoonsjebonden budget*—Keep the frail elderly at home as long as possible; reduce the demand for institutionalized care; reduce costs *Loopbaanonderbreking*—Create jobs; reduce unemployment
United Kingdom	Keep the frail elderly at home—*Community care* Stimulate the development of social networks Encourage the use of informal care *Attendants' Allowance*—To buy services *Invalid Care Allowance*—To provide some remuneration to the caregiver for the loss of income

Sources: Rostgaard and Fridberg, 1998; Jenson and Jacobzone, 2000.

response to perceived demographic and sociological shifts and to elderly persons' expressed preference for "aging in place" and followed from a desire to control public expenditure levels. Job creation and social solidarity goals were also important motives for policy makers.

As such, care allowance programs contribute to the redesign of welfare states and citizenship regimes. They do so by reinforcing a broader move toward marketization, which privileges market relations. Therefore, the market's portion of the welfare triangle increasingly dominates citizenship regimes in Europe, as it does elsewhere. In general, the arrival of neoliberalism in all types of welfare regimes has provoked a shift toward more flexible and diverse provision of services, under the rubric of valuing "choice." In this process, as Selma Sevenhuijsen argues in chapter 1, citizens become "consumers" of services and "clients" of the state, while the latter's role becomes one of maximizing choice. Marketization as a principle of social citizenship is now found in the social democratic welfare regime of Sweden, as well as in the more corporatist ones of continental Europe and the liberal regimes of North America.[21] Social citizenship as a meaningful construct may, as Sylvia Bashevkin suggests in chapter 5, be severely eroded and compromised as a result. With reference to care, the shift toward marketization is expressed in terms of substituting flexible systems for standardized ones, which in turn increases the diversity of programs, financing schemes, and provision arrangements.

Market forces are thus being introduced into a variety of relationships that previously were not marketized. Simultaneously, services that were both publicly financed and publicly provided are now being provided through markets, although not necessarily for profit, even when they are publicly financed. The marketization of informal care and homecare services provides an excellent example of this shift. Allowances paid to the frail elderly, as described in tables 3.1 and 3.2, are designed according to these principles of marketization. They are designed to increase citizens' "choice" and market capacity, albeit not always to the same extent. Table 3.1 documents how individuals may use the cash benefit to purchase services "in the market," whether from commercial or nonprofit providers or to "reimburse" their informal carers. Such a monetarization of relations blurs distinctions about market and nonmarket, about formal and informal, and about public and private provision. A second type of allowance is paid directly to carers, to "compensate" for lost income or for the costs of care. Carers are then able to use this income as a way to enter the labor market, in particular to benefit from labor market status with respect to social security regimes.

Care Allowances, Marketization, and Gender Relations

We have argued earlier and elsewhere that citizenship regimes in many European countries contained a commitment through the 1970s to gender equality, particularly with respect to employment.[22] This does not mean, of course, that gender equality existed, since that was clearly not the case. Nonetheless, the principle of promoting gender equality was one of several widely shared notions. Social movements and political formations subscribed to it, and the institutional machinery of the state at least in part promoted it.

This principle is now under threat from a number of directions. For example, an ideological commitment to the value of "choice" underlines a shift from commitment to equality of condition or results to a stance in favor of equality of opportunity. This move is visible in the citizenship regimes of Third Way governments, as examined by Sylvia Bashevkin in chapter 5. With attention turning to equality of opportunity, the "choices" made within families or by individual adult women (in contrast to girls or employers, who are still subject to the rules of "equal opportunity") are defined as resting beyond the responsibility of the state. A second example comes from public policy toward labor markets. Increasingly, states have accepted employers' claims that the "common conditions" imposed by postwar labor relations must be replaced by flexibility in labor markets, in which both employers and employees can "choose" their conditions of work, including the mix of full and part time and their individual labor contracts (see Leah F. Vosko's discussion in chapter 7). The result has been a generalized acceptance of part-time work, as well as of variation in labor contracts, as a characteristic of labor markets.[23]

These values inscribed in citizenship regimes in general have also shaped the gender dimension of care for the dependent elderly (see table 3.3). Most obviously, the frail elderly are being empowered as consumers with the capacity to choose. France's dependency allowance known as the PSD, Germany's dependency insurance, Austria's care allowances, and British attendant or carers' allowances, among others, all permit choice about care. Of course, some countries permit more choice than others. Germany sets no limits on expenditures, although it tilts the incentives in the direction of purchased services. France, in contrast, circumscribes who can be paid from the allowance and oversees the purchasing of services. Thus, the French citizenship regime is marketized, but the market is tightly controlled. Germany, Austria, and other countries with care allowances have, by way of contrast, tended to express greater confidence in the market behavior of their citizens.

Table 3.3: Consequences of Payments for Care for Women Who Are Caregivers

General Conclusions:

- Payments for care do not induce caregivers to withdraw from the labor market.
- Decisions are made on the basis of the needs of the frail elderly person.
- Payments for care do create jobs, but such employment is "atypical."
- Even when the frail elderly use formal services, they continue to use informal ones.

	A Gendered Benefit	The Work/Family "Balance"	Results for the Formal Care Sector and Women in the Labor Force
Germany	97% of caregivers with recognized status are women.	• Many caregivers are already retired, resulting in a heavy work load for the "healthy elderly." • Payments for care do provide a professional status, albeit parttime.	• Increase in demand for formal services. • Professionalization of some informal care work.
Austria	80% of those caring for someone receiving a care allowance are women.	• The payment for care "allowed" some caregivers to reduce their hours of employment.	• Less involvement of the voluntary sector in caring for the frail elderly.
Finland	80% of caregivers are women.		• Recipients combine formal and informal services.
France	Women hold 97% of personal service positions.		• Reduced black market employment. • Increase in atypical forms of employment. • Promotion of a market in personal services.

Source: Jenson and Jacobzone, 2000.

These design characteristics mean that the range of alternatives is significantly expanded. If the past menu was limited to institutional or familial care, then the present one aims to make more choices available. For frail elderly people—a great many of whom are women—this increase in choice is interpreted as giving greater "market power."

The question then becomes, How is market power used? Here the story is varied. Preliminary studies show that in some cases, an increase occurs in the consumption of formal services. This shift has consequences for women workers. In Germany, where a new professional category was created to accompany care insurance, the number of registered care workers rose. The story in the Netherlands is similar. However, it is also clear that the jobs being professionalized are low-paid, often part-time ones. These positions are often occupied by married women or other older women returning to the labor force. They are not generating economic autonomy in the classic sense, but are giving women who previously did not have it access to the labor market. In other words, work that in the past was done for free, either as informal family care or as volunteer work, is being marketized.

A similar process of transformation of informal work into market work, both paid and recognized by social security systems, is visible in countries that pay allowances to carers. In Finland, Austria, and Germany, care providers working with a family member may join pension and other regimes, thereby accumulating access to social benefits. Family caring has also acquired professional status in these cases. Therefore, whether the care provider is working inside the family or caring for an elderly person who is not a family member, payments for care include a market dimension. The carers are, in some cases, receiving money and in all cases are able to develop or maintain a link to some of the social benefits associated with labor market participation.

It must be stressed that the market relationship thus created is very limited in terms of income and accumulated rights. Nonetheless, it is worth noting as an analytic conclusion that both marketization and flexibilization of labor markets as principles have transformed informal and voluntary sector work into paid and protected work in these citizenship regimes.

The other dimension of care allowances that merits attention is the effect on the family economy. In many countries (including France, with the exception of spouses), payments for care can be used to "compensate" family members or can be accessed by family members. Therefore, the effect on the family economy in terms of internal transfers merits some attention. In some cases, the allowances were designed so that a frail elderly person could establish a contractual relationship with a care-provider.[24] In cases such as France, where a family member (but not a spouse) may be hired and the program demands a contract, the relationship must be under a contract. In Germany and Austria, however, where there are no limits on who can be "hired," there is very little evidence that such contractual relationships have actually been introduced into the family, especially between spouses or with children. When the allowance is not spent on services or to meet other costs, it tends to be absorbed into the general family budget or to be saved.

Thus far, then, marketization does not appear to be extending to the internal family economy, except to the extent that it is required, as in France. Gender relations as a result remain relatively unchanged. The allowance does little to guarantee economic self-sufficiency to the care-providers, who are treated as if they were "working for free," despite the existence of the allowance. Thus, the allowances in these cases have little effect on the amount of care designated as informal, both by the recipient and the provider.

Overall, then, care allowances hold mixed consequences. Because they tend to be paid at a low level, they help only the poorest among the frail elderly to reduce their economic dependency. Because care allowances are paid at a low level, they do not generate "good jobs" for the new "professions." Where recipients can decide how to spend the allowance, care payments do not seem to alter the principles of the family economy. High levels of informal care remain, and little income is transferred inside the family. On the other hand, payments for care do provide some measure of increased autonomy for elderly women, permitting them to avoid dependence on their families or institutionalization. Moreover, where such programs do recognize provision of care as "work," there is some integration of providers who were formerly in the informal or voluntary sector into the formal labor market, at least with respect to access to social benefits.

Thus, the story is a mixed one. On balance, however, marketization does not augur well for the achievement of real gender equality in the citizenship regimes-in-becoming. It is true that some unpaid work is being defined as "work" and therefore providing labor market benefits. Yet, at the same time, "work" itself is being further segmented. Gone is the idea of a single labor market, into which women might be incorporated as equals. Instead, we find a multiplication of labor markets, functioning according to a variety of rules. The market for care, whether home care or informal care, is one of these segments. The boundaries are blurred, as statuses shift and become hard to define. Whether one is "working" or "caring," paid or unpaid, is not always easy to assess.

While care allowances remain a work in progress, it is clear that the notion that most women would join a single labor market and have a relationship to it similar to men's no longer informs the citizenship regimes of Western Europe. Thus, the basic claim that animated so many women's movements of the second wave—that women must achieve economic autonomy in order to achieve equality—is again put into question.

Notes

This paper draws on earlier work reported in Jane Jenson and Stephane Jacobzone, *Care Allowances for the Frail Elderly and Their Impact on Women Care-givers* (OECD Labour Market and Social Policy Occasional Papers, no. 20, 2000). It extends, however, the coverage of European countries and does not consider non-European cases.

1. See Tine Rostgaard and Torben Fridberg, *Caring for Children and Older People—A Comparison of European Policies and Practices* (Copenhagen: Danish National Institute of Social Research, 1998), 50.
2. The classic formulation of this concept is presented in Gøsta Esping-Andersen, *The Three Worlds of Welfare Capitalism* (Princeton: Princeton University Press, 1990). For an influential feminist critique, see Ann Orloff, "Gender and the Social Rights of Citizenship: The Comparative Analysis of Gender Relations and Welfare States." *American Sociological Review* 58 (1993): 303–28.
3. This section is based on Jane Jenson, "Who Cares? Gender and Welfare Regimes," *Social Politics* 4 (1997): 182–87.
4. See OECD, *Caring for Frail Elderly People*, Social Policy Studies, no. 19; and Jenson and Jacobzone, *Care Allowances for the Frail Elderly*.
5. The concept was developed in Jane Jenson and Susan D. Phillips, "Regime Shift: New Citizenship Practices in Canada," *International Journal of Canadian Studies* 14 (1996): 111–35, in order to address issues of access to political institutions and processes of intermediation. It has also been applied to social policy restructuring in Jenson, "Who Cares?"; and in Gérard Boismenu and Jane Jenson, "A Social Union or a Federal State? Intergovernmental Relations in the New Liberal Era," in *How Ottawa Spends, 1998–99*, ed. Leslie Pal (Toronto: Oxford University Press, 1998), 57–79.
6. This offers an intervention in the growing literature on citizenship. In Will Kymlicka and Wayne Norman, "Return of the Citizen: A Survey of Recent Work on Citizenship Theory," in *Theorizing Citizenship*, ed. Ronald Beiner (Albany, N.Y.: SUNY Press, 1995), 283–322, the authors identified an "explosion of interest" in citizenship. Since they wrote this, interest continues unabated.
7. See Peter A. Hall and Rosemary C. R. Taylor, "Political Science and the Three New Institutionalisms," *Political Studies* 44 (1996): 936–57.
8. See Kathleen Thelen and Sven Steinmo, "Historical Institutionalism in Comparative Politics," in *Structuring Politics: Historical Institutionalism in Comparative Analysis*, by Sven Steinmo

et al. (New York: Cambridge University Press, 1992), 1–32; and Neil Bradford, *Commissioning Ideas: Canadian National Policy Innovation in Comparative Perspective* (Toronto: Oxford University Press, 1998).

9. For an English-language account of the regulation approach, see Alain Noël, "Accumulation, Regulation, and Social Change: An Essay on French Political Economy," *International Organization* 41 (1987): 303–33.
10. See also Kymlicka and Norman, "Return of the Citizen." Even in Canada, with its liberal welfare state, the emphasis was on equity, with a goal of overcoming structural blockages to fair and even equal participation (see Jenson and Phillips, "Regime Shift").
11. Kymlicka and Norman, "Return of the Citizen," 285–86.
12. For instance, as Shafir writes in his introduction to a reader on citizenship, "Citizenship, then, is an intellectual and moral tradition that has been repeatedly revisited and updated and, therefore, consists of a string of citizenship discourses." See Gershon Shafir, Introduction to *The Citizenship Debates: A Reader*, ed. Gershon Shafir (Minneapolis: University of Minnesota Press, 1998), 2.
13. See, for example, ibid., 23ff.
14. Stephan Leibfried and Paul Pierson, "Introduction," in *European Social Policy: Between Fragmentation and Integration*, ed. Stephan Leibfried and Paul Pierson (Washington, D.C.: Brookings Institution, 1995), 3.
15. For an overview of these issues, see the symposium on unpaid work and care in *Social Politics: International Studies in Gender, State, and Society*, vol. 4, no. 2. Indeed, that journal has had a watching brief on this issue from its inception.
16. The Nordic countries were something of an exception, since institutionalized care was provided as a social citizenship right. See J. Sipilä and A. Anttonnen, "Payments for Care: The Case of Finland," in *Payments for Care*, ed. Adalbert Evers, Marja Pilj, and Clare Ungerson (Aldershot: Avebury, 1994), 51–66; and Susan Christopherson, *Childcare and Elderly Care: What Occupational Opportunities for Women?* OECD Labour Market and Social Policy Occasional Papers, no. 27 (1997), 23.
17. See OECD, *Caring for Frail Elderly People*, 33.
18. See Kari Waerness and S. Ringen, "Women in the Welfare State: The Case of Formal and Informal Old-Age Care," in *The Scandinavian Model: Welfare States and Welfare Research*, by R. Erikson et al. (Armonk, N.Y.: M. E. Sharpe, 1987), 161–73.
19. Ibid., 169.
20. See Rostgaard and Fridberg, *Caring for Children and Older People*, 29.
21. See Jenson and Phillips, "Regime Shift"; Boismenu and Jenson, "A Social Union or a Federal State"; Jane Jenson and Mariette Sineau, *Qui doit garder le jeune enfant? Le travail des mères dans une Europe en crise* (Paris: L. G. D. J., 1997); and Julia S. O'Connor, Ann Shola Orloff, and Sheila Shaver, *States, Markets, Families: Gender,*

Liberalism, and Social Policy in Australia, Canada, Great Britain, and the United States (Cambridge: Cambridge University Press, 1999).
22. See, for example, Jenson and Sineau, *Qui doit garder le jeune enfant?*, chap. 10.
23. See Jane Jenson, Margaret Maruani, and Jacqueline Laufer, eds., *The Gendering of Inequalities: Women, Men, and Work* (Aldershot: Ashgate, 2000).
24. In Finland, the contract is between the municipal government and the care-provider, although the allowance is awarded to the person in need.

Part III
Anglo-American Welfare Reform

4.
Poverty, Social Assistance, and the Employability of Mothers in Four Commonwealth Countries

Maureen Baker

Introduction

In recent decades, governments in Anglo-American welfare states have restructured social programs in a way that asserts the primacy of markets over the state. Considerable research indicates that since about 1980, governments in countries such as Canada, Australia, New Zealand, the United Kingdom, and the United States have shifted toward a more residual and moralistic state that focuses on need, individual responsibility, and work incentives.[1]

During the 1970s in particular, social policy discourse in these countries placed greater emphasis than it subsequently did on social citizenship and universality. A more punitive approach to social program beneficiaries coincided since the 1980s with economic globalization and the international spread of neoliberalism as a major organizing theme of public policy. In justifying welfare state restructuring, government officials often claim that they are modernizing social programs and promoting program effectiveness. Yet many researchers argue that restructuring has been designed instead to reduce public expenditures, stimulate international investment, limit government deficits, and offer voters lower taxes.[2]

This chapter is based on the results of a larger cross-national study of restructuring in four major Commonwealth countries—Canada, Australia, New Zealand, and the United Kingdom—with a focus on programs for low-income mothers.[3] The project, funded by Human Resources Development Canada, involved travel to the four countries from 1996 to 1998 to examine policy documents, ministerial statements, government statistics, and empirical and theoretical studies of restructuring. A major concern of this study was to specify the macrolevel processes and outcomes of social program restructuring as they affect low-income mothers. Gender and maternal status are central analytic elements in the study, along with social class and political institutions. Since we based our research on four national case studies, we have been able to draw some broad conclusions about the discourse of restructuring and the impact of program reform on low-income mothers in liberal welfare states.

Restructuring in Liberal Welfare States

Esping-Andersen and others have classified all four countries in this study as liberal welfare regimes because government benefits have historically been relatively ungenerous, targeted to the poor, and funded through general taxation.[4] Yet substantial variations distinguish these cases from each other.[5] First, Canada and Australia are both federal systems in which policies are designed and administered by different levels of government, while New Zealand and Britain are unitary states. Second, Canada was established as a bicultural country with two languages and legal systems, while the other three countries are based primarily on English-language, common law traditions. Each country, with the exception of the United Kingdom, has a significant aboriginal population; all four are more culturally diverse over time, given high rates of immigration from Asia and elsewhere and, in the case of New Zealand, growing recognition of a vital Maori presence.

Third, numerous differences exist in the structure and practices of their governments. For example, New Zealand has a unicameral parliament and, since 1996, a proportional representation electoral system, while Canada has a bicameral federal parliament and a single member plurality electoral system. Fourth, a social insurance approach to unemployment insurance was used in Canadian and British social policy, while Australia and New Zealand relied mainly on regulation of the labor market and economy to create what was termed a "wage-earner's welfare state." Noticeable differences were also evident in the focus and pace of welfare state restructuring across these cases. Nevertheless, all four countries share many similarities in their cultural background, colonial past, legal system, and language, with the exception of Quebec in Canada, where the French language and civil law tradition are dominant.

In all four countries, entitlement to social benefits since the 1980s became increasingly conditional on the recipient's willingness to retrain for, search for, and obtain paid work. Paid work is regarded to varying degrees as morally superior to receiving benefits and tends to be less costly for governments.[6] In addition, moving people off social benefits has, as Sylvia Bashevkin argues in chapter 5, become more important than reducing poverty or assisting parents to combine paid work and family life. Consequently, official state rhetoric about social program eligibility has shifted away from citizenship rights, which imply some degree of permanent entitlement, toward a view of social benefits as temporary and designed to encourage self-sufficiency and labor market attachment. In the process, as Gwendolyn Mink and Leah F. Vosko demonstrate in part IV of this volume, structural barriers to unemployment and social rights to benefits no longer form a predominant part of government discourse.

In 1980 and following, government programs for low-income mothers began to rely directly on the labor market, private agencies, and the family for social provision. All four countries tightened their enforcement of child-support payments as a way to reduce social spending and enforce parental responsibility. They added user fees for health services and postsecondary education and tightened eligibility rules for social assistance programs. They linked social assistance, as well as unemployment benefits, to work incentives, skills training, and work tests. Yet restructuring efforts involved more than just cutbacks. Some governments actually improved social benefits for certain segments of the population, while they cut in other areas. In each country, elements of both consistency and contradiction occurred in the discourse concerning restructuring and employability. The policy outcomes for women were often fragmented, in that they advanced and retarded inequality at the same time.[7]

The pace and focus of change also differed across the four countries. The British government, for example, retained universal child benefits (although it froze their value for long periods) at the same time as other governments transformed universal family allowances into means-tested benefits. While some Canadian provinces and New Zealand cut basic rates of social assistance, Australia raised welfare payments and added new benefits. Canada encouraged low-income mothers into the workforce earlier than did the other countries, whether measured by the date of legislative change or the age of the youngest child. Australian politicians emphasized the importance of women's caring work at home more than their counterparts did in Canada.

In the four countries, the elevation of paid work and labor markets has been interpreted somewhat differently and has held varying policy consequences, especially when applied to low-income mothers. A substantial part of the explanation for this lies in national variations in economic and labor market trends, the varying strength of interest groups and their alignment with government, variations in the politics and structure of decision-making, and different ideas about families inherent in social programs. Each of these factors is addressed in the following sections.

Variations in the Treatment of Paid Work

Culturally specific models of family, motherhood, and the role of the state in family life underpin laws and social programs.[8] When the British established their colonies, they brought with them common law traditions and the idea that the state should intervene in family life only as a last resort. Although local pressures established varied practices, the tenor of social debates in Commonwealth countries remained heavily influenced by British policy ideas. At the turn of the century, British social programs were based on the male breadwinner model and the family wage, which preserved male work rights and weakened the right of married women to work, especially in times of high unemployment.[9] Furthermore, this approach encouraged a system of unemployment benefits that viewed wives as dependents, rather than as unemployed individuals, and paid married men benefits at a higher rate than unmarried men or women.

The institutionalization of the male breadwinner model into British social policy reinforced traditional notions about women's place long after families and labor markets had changed. Men tended to support this model because it allowed them to devote their attention to paid work with little concern about housework and child care. Governments endorsed the model because they were not obliged to provide expensive pay equity programs, maternity benefits, or public child-care services. Both men and women felt that children needed their mothers at home, and few alternative forms of care existed.[10] Yet as more women entered postsecondary education and paid work in the 1960s and following, the family wage eroded along with traditional gender role norms.

The family wage, however, was never institutionalized in Canada to the same degree that it was embedded in union agreements in Australia[11] and New Zealand and in social programs in the United Kingdom. This distinction in Canadian public policy was probably due more to structural than ideological variables, including the relative political weakness of labor unions in North America generally. As well, since the 1940s, Canadian unemployment insurance schemes were based on individual rather than family entitlement, as were old age pensions since 1951. Individual entitlement also became the basis from which Canadian feminist groups demanded employment reforms that recognized women as individuals (and employees), as well as dependents (and mothers).

By way of contrast, the United Kingdom, New Zealand, and especially Australia retained a stronger tradition of social benefits for mothering at home, based on the male breadwinner model. In Australia, additional government assistance for people who cared for children and the frail elderly at home was widely supported throughout the 1990s, at a time when benefits were being cut in other jurisdictions.[12] In New Zealand, new workfare programs were introduced in 1998, but the Domestic Purposes Benefit continued to be paid to parents until their youngest child was fourteen years old. Nevertheless, beneficiaries whose youngest child was aged seven to fourteen were expected to seek part-time work or community service placements after 1998.

In Britain, a discrepancy in public discourse became apparent over time. Beginning in 1997, the New Labour government encouraged lone mothers to participate in New Deal welfare-to-work programs, citing the relative poverty and lower employment rates among this group than among partnered mothers (see Sylvia Bashevkin's discussion in chapter 5). Nevertheless, Labour government policy documents refer to "second earners" when speaking of wives in two-earner families, thus reflecting an updated formulation of the male breadwinner model.[13]

Low-income mothers' greater involvement in paid work requires policies promoting the affordability and availability of child care. More than the other countries, Canada has recognized the link between subsidized child care and employment opportunities for mothers. Australia, Britain, and New Zealand still treat child care more as an educational issue than as a support for working parents. Furthermore, employability schemes in the four countries fail to address the gendered division of labor within households, where wives and mothers are not absolved of their caring responsibilities. Instead, as Selma Sevenhuijsen and Jane Jenson suggest with reference to Western Europe in chapters 1 and 3, women are encouraged to better manage their double burden of paid work and unpaid care. Nevertheless, until gendered inequalities within the home are resolved, women will continue to be at a competitive disadvantage in paid employment.

Economic and Labor Market Trends

Restructuring in all four countries has also occurred in a context of globalization, growing concern about government debt and deficits, rising social expenditures as a percentage of gross domestic product, and unemployment levels that contribute to social program costs.[14] These economic constraints, however, have not been interpreted by all governments in the same way.

The relationship between debt levels, politics, and social programs is striking. As table 4.1 indicates, both Canada and New Zealand experienced comparatively high government debt levels relative to gross domestic product, especially after 1985. Resolving the "debt crisis" became a major political issue in both cases,

Table 4.1: Government Debt as Percentage of GDP, 1980–1995

Year	Canada	Australia	New Zealand	United Kingdom
1980	44.3	24.9	50.6	54.0
1985	64.1	26.2	72.9	58.9
1990	72.5	21.3	59.7	39.3
1995	99.1	43.8	50.9	57.6

Source: OECD economic surveys, 1980–1995.

creating opportunities for manipulative politics and selective budget cuts. Only Canada and New Zealand actually cut social benefit levels, yet the overall level of social security paid by both governments in 1995 as a percentage of GDP remained higher than in the other two countries (see table 4.2). Foreign leaders and employers' groups pressured the New Zealand Labour government in the 1980s to refinance the debt, float the currency, open the country to foreign investment, and reduce government spending. The dramatic changes that followed had not been anticipated by many New Zealanders who voted for Labour and led to considerable debate about the country's "Great Experiment" in economic restructuring. Concern over Canada's high public debt permeated most political parties through the 1990s. Canada's national debt was relatively high, and high unemployment rates were also viewed as a major political concern.

From the 1940s to the 1960s, neither Australia nor New Zealand developed expansive social programs, but relied instead on high

Table 4.2: Government Social Security Benefits as Percentage of GDP, 1960–1995

Date	Canada	Australia	New Zealand	United Kingdom
1960	8.0	5.5	–	6.1
1970	8.1	5.5	–	8.0
1980	10.1	9.1	–	10.6
1990	13.2	10.5	17.5	10.7
1995	14.9	13.0	15.7	13.7

Source: Baker and Tippin, 1999, 31.

wages and state protection of labor and markets for income security. Both countries reported a fairly small gap between the earnings of rich and poor men at the beginning of the 1980s, compared to other OECD nations with more generous social programs and lower poverty rates.[15] Yet this dispersion grew throughout the 1980s as unemployment rose and as Labour governments in both countries decentralized wage bargaining and cut some social programs. By the 1990s, New Zealand had reduced its highest marginal tax rate to 33 percent, while Australia kept its rate at 49 percent. New Zealand dropped many protective tariffs, introduced a goods and services tax, and reduced social benefits, while Australia did not. Consequently, the gap between rich and poor widened faster in New Zealand than in Australia.[16]

Both New Zealand and several Canadian provinces cut welfare payments at a time when Australia was improving health-care coverage and increasing benefits for caring work. Furthermore, Australia, New Zealand, and the United Kingdom retained social benefits for low-income mothers caring for school-aged children at home. In contrast, many Canadian provinces expected mothers to enter the paid workforce when their youngest child reached school age or before, as table 4.3 indicates.

Our research suggests that providing a long-term social benefit for mothering at home is one factor that inhibits the paid

Table 4.3: Employability Requirements for Mothers on Social Assistance by Age of Youngest Child, 1998

Country	Age of Youngest Child
Canada	Alberta: 6 months
	Quebec, Yukon: 2 years
	Ontario: 3–6 years
	Manitoba: 6 years
	British Columbia: 7 years
Australia	16 years
New Zealand	14 years
United Kingdom	16 years

Source: Baker and Tippin, 1999, 243.

employment of mothers. Canadian lone mothers, who have less official encouragement for mothering at home than their counterparts in the other three cases, are more than twice as likely as New Zealand and British lone mothers to be employed full time (see table 4.4). In the absence of social benefits, full-time employment offers the possibility, but not necessarily the actuality, of self-support, since the chances of self-sufficiency based on part-time earnings are minimal without additional government or family funds. Until 1996, Canadian welfare rules discouraged part-time work by allowing only very limited earnings before social assistance was withdrawn. Following the establishment of the Canada Health and Social Transfer in 1996, most provinces permitted beneficiaries to work part time and receive partial benefits, but some, including Ontario, as discussed in Leah F. Vosko's chapter, created punitive workfare programs.

The paid employment of lone mothers is also influenced by divorce rates, fertility trends, and legal responsibilities. Marriage dissolution leads to greater economic uncertainty for all family members, but especially for mothers who retain custody of their children. Canada has the highest divorce rate of the four countries under consideration, but most Canadian women believe they need to earn a living, regardless of marital or parental status.[17] Higher rates of paid employment fit well with low fertility, and Canadian women have the lowest fertility rates of the four countries.[18] Furthermore, Canadian family law specifies that mothers, as well as fathers, must support their children.[19]

Among lone mothers, levels of reliance on social assistance benefits are the highest in Australia and the lowest in Canada, but the

Table 4.4: Percentage of Mothers in Full- and Part-Time Employment, 1994–95

	Single Mothers			Partnered Mothers		
	Employed	F-T	P-T	Employed	F-T	P-T
Canada	57	32	25	74	41	33
Australia	43	22	21	51	27	24
New Zealand	27	17	10	58	31	27
United Kingdom	41	17	24	62	22	40

Source: Baker and Tippin, 1999, 29.

discourse critical of "welfare dependency" seems to be less pronounced in Australia than in the other cases. Typically, the Australian emphasis is on mothers' caring responsibilities and their "choice" of caring over paid work. Most lone mothers in Australia, New Zealand, and Britain depend partially or entirely on government benefits, rather than on paid work. About 94 percent of Australian, 89 percent of New Zealand, and 79 percent of U.K. single mothers rely on social assistance, compared to only 44 percent of Canadian lone mothers.[20] Despite this comparatively low rate in Canada, the prevailing discourse in that country contends that "welfare dependency" is too high, welfare rules are outmoded, and more work incentives are needed. Comparative North American research by Sylvia Bashevkin (chapter 5) and Leah F. Vosko (chapter 7) in this volume suggests Canada's close geographic proximity to the United States may be a crucial factor in explaining differences between Canada and other Commonwealth countries in this respect.

Wage levels and the value of social benefits are also important to compare. As table 4.5 indicates, net disposable monthly income after housing costs for both two- and one-parent families on benefits in 1992 was the highest in Australia and the lowest in New Zealand. After 1992, benefits were reduced in several Canadian provinces, which made net disposable income in Canada close to New Zealand levels. Canada also ranked poorly in terms of the value of social assistance relative to wages, especially after housing costs were included, as table 4.6 indicates.

Table 4.5: Net Disposable Monthly Income of Families on Social Benefits, 1992

Country	Before Housing Costs		After Housing Costs	
	1-Parent Families	2-Parent Families	1-Parent Families	2-Parent Families
Canada	806	909	481	585
Australia	677	951	544	758
New Zealand	628	742	380	472
United Kingdom	506	639	499	626

Source: Baker and Tippin 1999, 35.

Note: Families are defined here as parent(s) aged 35, with one child who was 3 years of age. All amounts are reported in U.S. dollars.

Table 4.6: Social Assistance Rates for Families with One 7-Year-Old Child, as Percentage of Net Disposable Income at Average Earnings, 1992

Country	Before Housing Costs		After Housing Costs	
	Lone Parent with 1 Child	Couple with 1 Child	Lone Parent with 1 Child	Couple with 1 Child
Canada	42	47	36	44
Australia	44	60	47	64
New Zealand	49	58	42	54
United Kingdom	32	42	37	49

Source: Baker and Tippin 1999, 35.

Our study indicates that social assistance does not raise people above a subsistence or poverty line in all countries, especially those such as Canada and New Zealand that cut benefit levels in the 1990s. We also conclude that economic security for low-income mothers on benefits is not guaranteed by paid employment. The Canadian case is quite revealing in this respect. Canada has the highest paid labor force participation rates for women of the four countries considered, and significantly more women there are employed full time. Yet the incidence of low-paid employment in Canada, for both men and women, is greater than in the other three countries.[21] Indeed, the high incidence of low-paid work for Canadian men (16.1 percent in 1994, compared to 11.8 percent in Australia) helps to explain high rates of employment for women. Canadian mothers worked for pay in large part because male wages fell and manufacturing jobs disappeared under global trade agreements at the same time that the cost of living increased rapidly. As well, Canadian unions were less effective in protecting wages than were Australian unions. Therefore, a second income became essential to maintain living standards even in two-parent households in Canada.

In Australia, New Zealand, and Britain, by way of contrast, mothers were marginalized in the workforce by structural constraints. Both Australia and New Zealand lack statutory maternity benefits, although paid maternity leave is available to many unionized workers. Affordable and high-quality child care is hard to find in all three countries; moreover, fees are particularly high in Britain and New Zealand.[22] In the absence of statutory maternity benefits and public child care, many women in Australia and New Zealand leave the labor force after childbirth and find it difficult to return. Yet cultural values still encourage women in these countries to view themselves primarily as homemakers and mothers and therefore to forgo the job training or work experience necessary to find well-paying positions. Low-income mothers thus face serious obstacles to earning a living wage.

Variations in Interest Group Mobilization

Powerful constituencies of support have developed over the years for existing social programs, including among trade unions and feminist organizations. In all four countries, the labor movement played a central role in the development of social programs that privileged employed men and consigned women to a role as men's dependents. In some cases, the family wage model became integrated into labor market policy and social programs precisely because trade unions wanted to protect male workers.[23] In Australia and New Zealand, unions persuaded governments to control prices and restrict foreign competition and labor in order to protect local jobs, inflate wages, and enable high rates of home ownership.[24] The family wage was thus institutionalized through a centralized system of wage fixing and arbitration in Australia, New Zealand, and the United Kingdom.

North American unions supported the family wage concept early in the twentieth century because it maintained high male wages and excluded cheap female and foreign labor.[25] Yet the weakness of the North American labor movement, with no history of centralized bargaining, meant Canadian organizations could not maintain the family wage position. Since the 1980s, the Canadian labor movement has been challenged by efforts to restrict employment rights and to introduce free-trade agreements, technological change, and growing numbers of part-time workers, who are difficult to organize. Moreover, most Canadian unions allied themselves at the federal level with the New Democratic party, a formation that has yet to win power at that level.

In Australia, economic restructuring was negotiated through quasi-corporatist agreements between unions and government during the 1980s. This process produced relatively gradual reforms that protected earnings and the social wage. In contrast, the New Zealand government pushed through quick reforms with little public discussion and generated widespread protest. Yet centralized bargaining eroded over time in both countries. Union membership declined sharply, especially in New Zealand,[26] thus weakening labor movement influence and strengthening the role of business groups.

Although mainstream welfare state theorists downplay the influence of women's groups in developing and reforming social policy, feminist researchers have underlined their importance.[27] Early in the twentieth century, feminists opposed the family wage system and were instrumental in pressing for public education, family allowances, maternity benefits, income assistance, and child-care services.[28] In Anglo-American countries, women remain over-represented as employees and clients of social welfare agencies and have often used this status to argue for continued state provision.

Canadian women's groups were generally more cohesive and influential in public policy debates than were women's movements in the other three countries. In 1970, the Royal Commission on the Status of Women in Canada successfully recommended the creation of both an advisory council and a federal government department devoted to improving women's position. Since then, various interest groups consisting predominantly of women successfully demanded paid national maternity benefits, pay equity policies, and subsidies for child-care.[29] Although some efforts were made to lobby for a homemaker's wage, these were less successful than campaigns for employment rights in the regular labor force.[30]

British feminism was not particularly successful in promoting either women's employment rights or individual entitlement to social benefits. Vicky Randall argues that feminist mobilization around child care achieved less since 1970 in Britain than in other English-speaking countries.[31] She attributes this to a number of factors, including the movement's fragmentation by ideology and social class, changing views about the relevance of children to the women's movement, concerns that state-run child care would perpetuate patriarchy and capitalism, and disagreements over how parenting and employment for mothers should be organized.

More women were brought into elite positions under the New Labour government since 1997 than during previous Conservative regimes, but feminist priorities often seemed tangential to public policy debates during the Blair years.[32] Women activists accused both Conservative and Labour parties of using the rhetoric of feminism without much substance, or "equal opportunism."[33] They also criticized Labour for its focus on "family values" and "unbounded individualism," both of which recall values promoted by the Conservatives. British feminists, therefore, questioned whether New Labour would dramatically improve social policies for women.

Women's groups met with varying degrees of success in achieving gender equity and protecting their policy gains. They pursued varied objectives, from an emphasis on "choices" to enter paid work with public assistance to one that would support mothers to remain at home. Major differences appear across political systems. In Canada, the policy environment favored paid employment and working mothers, offered government support for child care and paid maternity leave, and provided an equality clause in the federal constitution that was absent in the other three countries. By way of contrast, cultural legacies in Australia, Britain, and New Zealand elevated motherhood and caring to the status of national icons, and widely regarded public child care with suspicion.[34] These legacies limited the vigor with which women's groups could pursue issues related to paid work and child care.

Employer groups have long formed powerful lobbies in these four countries and were particularly influential in recent years. In Canada and New Zealand, concerns over high public debts, combined with a weak political left, provided fertile ground for conservatives to exercise stronger influence over public policy. Business groups cannot be considered vigorous advocates for women's interests; instead, they have lobbied for lower taxes, reduced public spending, and less government regulation of the market. Business lobbies were also major actors in the "welfare dependency" debate. In New Zealand, they helped to overturn broadly supported social policies in the 1980s and 1990s and pushed for the 1998 workfare program and a proposed Code of Social and Family Responsibility, which emphasized greater individual and family responsibility for income security and well-being.[35]

The pervasiveness of pro-market philosophies across political parties in the four countries is noteworthy. In Australia and New Zealand, center-left parties initiated state restructuring and took some tentative steps toward bringing social benefits recipients closer to the market. New Zealand's center-right government was in the process of moving employability schemes to the forefront when Labour won the 1999 election. The Australian center-right government proceeded somewhat more cautiously. In the United Kingdom, as discussed by Sylvia Bashevkin in the next chapter, New Labour launched a series of New Deal schemes to bring more people into paid employment, thus operationalizing some of the older rhetoric of Thatcherite Conservatives. This pattern indicates that an emphasis on employability is not the exclusive property of any political party or any specific location on the left-right spectrum.

In Canada, much of the political activity related to employability occured at the provincial level and cut across the spectrum. Yet the pattern at the national level suggested some parallels to Britain: The federal Conservative party in Canada set the ideological tone for employability discussions during its tenure, and this focus was consolidated by a federal Liberal party that was traditionally viewed as center-left. While we do not want to overemphasize convergence across the four countries, the degree of political consensus within each case is impressive and typically found only in such realms as foreign policy.

The degree to which each political culture tolerates a permanent underclass is also important in explaining the uneven path of restructuring. Canada's proximity to the United States, with its means-tested welfare system and workfare programs, appears to lead to greater Canadian tolerance of not only a growing category of disadvantaged working poor, but also sustained reliance on food banks and homeless people sleeping in the streets. On the other hand, the Australian emphasis on giving all citizens a "fair go" seems to moderate more radical, pro-market tendencies.

Decision-Making and the Structure of Government

Power resource theorists argue that the structure of government can influence the speed and extent of restructuring.[36] A nation with one central government can make rapid decisions, while a federation may require time-consuming consultations in order to reach a national consensus. Yet a centralized government may also delay policy reforms, while state or provincial governments can pressure federal governments to act more rapidly. A bicameral parliamentary system requires legislation to pass through two decision-making units, which takes more time and effort than passing policy through a unicameral system. In addition, an electoral system based on first-past-the-post rules sometimes allows one party to gain a majority of seats, even when most voters in the country choose other parties. This means that policies opposed by smaller parties can still be passed into law. And finally, a government dominated by men, privileged socioeconomic classes, or one cultural group may pass legislation that does not represent the wishes of women, the working classes, or cultural minorities.

Our cross-national research reinforces the idea that the structure of government influences policy reform. New Zealand is the prime example of a nation that rapidly changed from state control over much of the economy to heavy reliance on foreign markets and the private sector. Within ten years, New Zealand dismantled its state and downsized social programs more rapidly and extensively than did other industrialized nations. This was facilitated by a unicameral system in which the cabinet dominated social and economic policy. No provincial or state governments could serve as institutional bases for opposition to government restructuring. Protests by the labor movement and community groups were weak, and the major political opposition—the Labour party—was compromised by its role as the initiator of reform in the 1980s. The result in New Zealand was that a small political/bureaucratic/business alliance with an ideologically coherent program effected a major policy overhaul.

Although the post-1996 proportional representation system in New Zealand was supposed to act as a political brake on rapid change, this arrangement did not prevent a conservative coalition government in 1998 from making extensive changes to social benefits. It did so within two days by introducing legislation under "urgency" provisions, thus bypassing extensive public hearings. Clearly, reforms to the electoral system, as occurred in New Zealand, do not necessarily slow the process of welfare state restructuring.

In contrast, Canadian federal government action is often limited by jurisdictional disputes and the necessity to consult with provincial governments. Despite constraints that follow from efforts to keep Quebec within the federation, the Liberal government reduced federal expenditures by changing federal/provincial social funding arrangements. As Sylvia Bashevkin and Leah F. Vosko argue in chapters 5 and 7, the establishment of the Canada Health and Social Transfer in 1996 allowed the federal government to save money while permitting more provincial control over social programs.

Subtle changes in political processes can also affect welfare state reform. Institutional reforms specific to each country can pressure against the maintenance of existing social programs. In New Zealand, ideologically inspired budget-cutters gained control over the treasury. As that department gained power over other bureaucratic structures, tax cuts (which diminished the state's revenue base) further undermined the future of some social programs. Moreover, the 1991 Employment Contracts Act weakened the ability of unions in New Zealand to act as advocates for welfare state programs.

Because women are major users of welfare programs and form the bulk of welfare state workers, the policy outcomes of these debates are highly gendered.[37] In particular, women have traditionally been marginalized from elite decision-making positions in all four countries,[38] and political norms have inhibited women's participation. Helga Hernes, Marilyn Waring, and others have argued that the involvement of women—or lack thereof—in government decision-making affects the evolution of social policy.[39] In their view, welfare state programs are often biased against women's interests in cases like the four under consideration, where women are far less numerous at elite levels than in Scandinavian countries, for example.

Theorizing Restructuring

Across welfare states, the needs and roles of low-income mothers have been conceptualized differently and policy reforms have varied. Yet in recent years, all four countries have adopted similar strategies that emphasize the paid employment of lone parents in order to restrict entitlement to social provision. This focus on employability devalues social provision, and, as Leah F. Vosko argues in chapter 7, it contains ideological assumptions about the importance of work discipline for beneficiaries.

As governments in all four countries questioned the basic tenets of the welfare state, they pressed hard on arguments against "welfare dependency." The ideological dominance of neoliberalism meant that alternative policy initiatives, including those proposed by Gwendolyn Mink and Leah F. Vosko in part IV of this volume, lacked political sponsorship. A variety of progressive policy options, such as government-sponsored job creation programs or a guaranteed annual income, were discredited as "politically unfeasible."

Labor market and economic trends also influenced the restructuring process. Labor surpluses were more common than labor shortages in some regions of the four countries. The low-wage end of employment markets was dramatically affected by the decline of manufacturing jobs and the rise of the service sector. Increasingly, the jobs available to many low-income mothers were insecure, were low paid, and involved weak statutory and union protections. In economies where ethnic and racial minorities were historically disadvantaged, the disappearance of traditional employment opportunities for these minorities constrained their ability to seek and retain paid work. Rapid urbanization and the cumulative impact of low educational attainment often compounded these effects.

Theories of restructuring must therefore include an assessment of women's labor force participation, which both influences and is influenced by policy decisions. In Canada, relatively high rates of full-time employment for mothers and the need for two family incomes created a strong constituency for public child care. In contrast, the demand for public child care remained much weaker in places where the male breadwinner model continued to reinforce the primary status of women as caregivers, rather than wage earners. Consequently, employability programs for lone mothers on social assistance in Australia, Britain, and New Zealand focused less attention on the mothers of preschool-age children.

Understanding welfare state reform in relation to low-income mothers also requires us to consider the gendered nature of family life, as incorporated into social programs. During the 1930s and following, patriarchal family models mirrored and perpetuated prevailing gender relations in the family and society. Historically, women in the four countries typically became social assistance beneficiaries through maternity or changes in their relationships with men, rather than through their labor force attachment.[40] Although economic, social, and demographic conditions changed over time, many social programs continued to portray partnered women as men's dependents and lone mothers as primarily mothers, rather than as potential employees. Among these four cases, social programs in Canada were the exception, since Canadian women moved more rapidly into full-time employment than did their Commonwealth counterparts and became recipients of work-related benefits, as well as of means-tested social assistance. Yet Canadian family law and new employability programs sometimes overestimated women's opportunities to become self-supporting, as they often did in the United States as well.

Understanding the process of reforming social provision means that gendered ideologies and practices about family and work must be acknowledged and analyzed. Much of women's work has been unpaid and related to caring activities within the home or within the community. Whether or not mothers enter the labor force relates to changing economic conditions, employment opportunities, family arrangements, and union agreements, but it is also linked to prevailing ideologies about women's capacities, children's needs, and the social acceptance of child care from sources outside the immediate family.

Conclusions

Mothers with preschool- and school-aged children typically enter and leave the labor force under different conditions than do most men. Women are more likely than men to work part time, to be employed in the public sector and in voluntary organizations, to accept clerical and service positions, and to hold low-paid, temporary, and nonunionized jobs. Positions in the public sector and voluntary organizations remain particularly vulnerable to cutbacks in countries whose governments are sympathetic to neoliberal ideologies. Furthermore, part-time job vacancies are in many cases growing faster than full-time ones, yet the former seldom lead to economic self-sufficiency. In short, low-income people, especially lone mothers and people from ethnic and racial minority backgrounds, frequently bear the brunt of economic restructuring.

Although some Anglo-American employability programs offered child-care services and opportunities for individual counseling, many participants were mothers with young children or persons with disabilities or illnesses, who found it difficult to enter a competitive labor force. If they could find and retain paid jobs and actually exit from poverty, then they required considerable assistance. Moreover, as Leah F. Vosko demonstrates in chapter 7, employability programs usually focused on individual-level educational achievement, employment skills, work habits, interviewing skills, and attitudes, instead of on structural barriers to market income. The latter would include the shortage of paid work in some communities, family responsibilities that often interfered with full-time employment, emotional or physical disabilities, and the availability of affordable child care. Furthermore, employability programs in Anglo-American countries tended to view rearing children as a family responsibility, rather than as a social obligation.

Employability programs were also designed to be gender-neutral. They assumed that the labor market treated all individuals equally and that gender, race, and class were irrelevant to unemployment or underemployment. In reality, however, men and women tend to compete in labor markets on unequal terms. Men typically participate as relatively unencumbered individuals and more closely approximate the "rational economic actors" of econometric models than do most mothers. Although employability programs excluded mothers with preschool-aged children in Australia, New Zealand, and the United Kingdom, these schemes were gradually being modified to include mothers with younger children in all four countries. The idea that all adults should become self-supporting wage earners with full-time jobs remains a less feasible notion for low-income mothers than for unemployed men or women without children. As Selma Sevenhuijsen suggests in chapter 1, trying to make all women into unencumbered economic actors without family roles not only lays the groundwork for policy failure, but also increases burdens upon women to manage both low-paid work and unpaid domestic responsibilities.

Gendering the concept of employability means acknowledging that drawing low-income people into paid work may hold different consequences for men and women. Attempts to make mothers more employable were strenuously resisted in countries such as Australia, New Zealand, and the United Kingdom, where mothers were expected to care for their own young children at home. In countries such as Canada, there was a broader acceptance of nonmaternal child care during the workday. In short, even as the official emphasis placed upon paid work for low-income mothers rose in all four countries, the devaluation of mothering at home and commodification of child care varied cross-nationally.

Enhancing the employability of low-income mothers involves an implicit attempt to reconstruct personal and social identities, including what it means to be a "good mother," carer, paid worker, and citizen. The identity reconstruction demanded by these schemes encourages mothers coming off social benefits to see themselves more as independent employees and less as family carers or volunteers. Yet, as Selma Sevenhuijsen and Jane Jenson ask in previous chapters, who will do the caring work in society if low-income women are pushed into the paid labor force? Low-income workers will not be able to afford high-quality child-care services without government subsidies. The supposed consensus that says that most social assistance beneficiaries want and should work for pay is thus more problematic than it initially appears.

Gender is incorporated into Anglo-American employability programs in at least two different ways. In Canada, a full-time worker/mother model of citizenship is supported in principle by modest levels of public child-care provision and constitutionally entrenched equality rights. In Australia, New Zealand, and the United Kingdom, the dominant model remains mother/part-time worker, reflecting a profound social ambivalence about mothers in the labor force and an emphasis on gender difference, rather than on gender equality.[41] The emphasis on mothers' part-time work, while retaining responsibility for caring, provides a convenient way for politicians in these countries to reconcile the neoliberal concept of employability with the policy legacy left by the male breadwinner model.

In all four cases, the evolving shape of social provision holds mixed prospects for alleviating poverty, especially among low-income mothers. Increased government attention will likely be directed toward the conditions of entry into paid work and the removal of barriers that make mothers reluctant workers. Social safety nets could be redesigned around periods between paid jobs and could provide reduced levels of income support for women who are deemed to be unemployable. To facilitate longer attachment to paid employment, improvements would be necessary in such areas as child care, statutory parental leave, and training and education. These reforms could represent an increased incorporation of gender considerations into social program design, but their potential impact is mitigated by at least three other factors.

First, low-income mothers with caring responsibilities can never fully conform to the "rational man" model that underpins employability programs. Second, employability is not the solution to poverty for all beneficiaries. Total incomes for some mothers might improve if they were able to earn income while receiving partial benefits, but this could be offset by low pay, insecure jobs in an unprotected labor market, and higher employment expenses. Since minimum wages rarely provide "living wages," and those receiving them have little power to negotiate their employment choices, paid work is not always the best path out of poverty. As Sylvia Bashevkin notes in the next chapter, however, employability programs could prove to be less about poverty than about a moralistic campaign against lone mothers. Finally, existing benefits for the poor might be targeted even more narrowly, fueled by strong political pressure in all four countries to reduce taxes.

Employability programs could offer a partial solution to poverty and reliance on benefits, but they do not address the problems of low-paid work, structural unemployment, and gender inequalities.

In fact, liberal welfare states may have reduced class inequality between the 1940s and the 1970s, but the poverty of low-income mothers and their children was not seriously challenged even during the expansionary phase of the four Commonwealth welfare states examined in this account. The outlook for reducing poverty during a period of economic growth and program contraction appears equally bleak. In this view, neither economic nor social well-being is guaranteed through paid work in an unfettered market. Moreover, the links between poverty, social assistance, and employability are deeply gendered and require gendered analytical approaches.

Finally, we need to acknowledge that policy changes are typically incremental. Different governments with varying agendas tend to amend existing programs, rather than impose sweeping reforms. This incrementalism, as well as the diverse situations of those relying on social provision, suggests that it may be worthwhile to probe specific programs or other microlevel aspects of welfare states, especially in cross-national research. In so doing, researchers need to use carefully nuanced conceptions of gender, work, and family in order to unravel the dynamics of changing social provision.

Notes

1. See Sylvia Bashevkin, *Women on the Defensive: Living through Conservative Times* (Chicago: University of Chicago Press, 1998); Maureen Baker and David Tippin, *Poverty, Social Assistance, and the Employability of Mothers: Restructuring Welfare States* (Toronto: University of Toronto Press, 1999); and Julia S. O'Connor, Ann Shola Orloff, and Sheila Shaver, *States, Markets, Families: Gender, Liberalism, and Social Policy in Australia, Canada, Great Britain, and the United States* (Cambridge: Cambridge University Press, 1999).
2. See Ramesh Mishra, *The Welfare State in Capitalist Society* (Toronto: University of Toronto Press, 1990); Paul Pierson, *Dismantling the Welfare State? Reagan, Thatcher, and the Politics of Retrenchment* (Cambridge: Cambridge University Press, 1994); Gøsta Esping-Andersen, ed., *Welfare States in Transition: National Adaptations in Global Economies* (London: Sage, 1996); John Myles, "When Markets Fail: Social Welfare in Canada and the United States," in *Welfare States in Transition*, ed. Esping-Andersen, 116–40; and Jonathan Boston, Paul Dalziel, and Susan St. John, *Redesigning the Welfare State in New Zealand* (Auckland: Auckland University Press, 1999).

3. See Baker and Tippin, *Poverty, Social Assistance, and the Employability of Mothers.*
4. See Gøsta Esping-Andersen, *The Three Worlds of Welfare Capitalism* (Cambridge: Polity Press, 1990).
5. See Deborah Mitchell, *Income Transfers in Ten Welfare States* (Aldershot: Avebury, 1991); Maureen Baker, *Canadian Family Policies: Cross-National Comparisons* (Toronto: University of Toronto Press, 1995); and Francis G. Castles, "Needs-Based Strategies of Social Protection in Australia and New Zealand," in *Welfare States in Transition*, ed. Esping-Andersen, 88–115.
6. See Ruth Lister, "Citizenship Engendered," in *Critical Social Policy*, ed. David Taylor (London: Sage, 1996), 168–74.
7. See Rosemary Du Plessis, "Stating the Contradictions: The Case of Women's Employment," in *Feminist Voices: Women's Studies Texts for Aotearoa/New Zealand* (Auckland: Oxford University Press, 1992), 209–23.
8. See Margrit Eichler, *Family Shifts: Families, Policies, and Gender Equality* (Toronto: Oxford University Press, 1997).
9. See Hilary Land, "The Family Wage," University of Leeds, Eleanor Rathbone Memorial Lecture, 1979; and Maureen Baker and Mary-Anne Robeson, "Trade Union Reactions to Women Workers and Their Concerns," *Canadian Journal of Sociology* 6 (1981): 19–31.
10. See Diane Sainsbury, *Gender, Equality, and Welfare States* (Cambridge: Cambridge University Press, 1996).
11. For example, the family wage was part of the Australian Arbitration Court's Harvester Agreement of 1907.
12. See Sheila Shaver, Anthony King, Marilyn McHugh, and Toni Payne, *At the End of Eligibility: Female Sole Parents Whose Youngest Child Turns 16* (Sydney, Australia: University of New South Wales, Social Policy Research Centre, Reports and Proceedings #117, 1994); and Bruce Bradbury, *Income Support for Parents and Other Carers* (Sydney: University of New South Wales, Social Policy Research Centre, 1996).
13. See United Kingdom, HM Treasury, *Financial Statement and Budget Report* (House of Commons Paper No. HC 62; London: The Stationary Office, 1998).
14. See Jane Kelsey, *Economic Fundamentalism* (London: Pluto Press, 1995); Castles, "Needs-Based Strategies of Social Protection in Australia and New Zealand"; and Myles, "When Markets Fail."
15. See Bruce Bradbury, "Male Wage Inequality before and after Tax: A Six Country Comparison," Discussion Paper #42, Social Policy Research Centre. Sydney: University of New South Wales, 1993.
16. See Francis G. Castles and Ian F. Shirley, "Labour and Social Policy: Gravediggers or Refurbishers of the Welfare State?" in *The Great Experiment: Labour Parties and Public Policy Transformation in Australia and New Zealand*, ed. F. Castles, R. Gerritsen, and J. Vowles (Auckland: Auckland University Press, 1996), 88–106.
17. See Baker and Tippin, *Poverty, Social Assistance, and the Employability of Mothers*, 27.

18. Ibid.
19. See Maureen Baker and Shelley Phipps, "Family Change and Family Policy: Canada," in *Family Change and Family Policies in Britain, Canada, New Zealand, and the United States*, ed. Sheila Kamerman and Alfred Kahn (Oxford: Oxford University Press, 1997), 103–206.
20. Compare data in Jonathan Bradshaw, Steven Kennedy, Majella Kilkey, Sandra Hutton, Anne Corden, Tony Eardley, Hilary Holmes, and Joanne Neale, *Policy and Employment of Lone Parents in 20 Countries* (Brussels: Commission of the European Communities, 1996), 52; with those in Martin Dooley, "Lone-Mother Families and Social Assistance Policy in Canada," in *Family Matters: New Policies for Divorce, Lone Mothers, and Child Poverty*, by Martin Dooley et al. (Toronto: C. D. Howe Institute, 1995), 35–104.
21. Low-paid employment is defined here as less than two-thirds of the median wage for full-time workers. See Baker and Tippin, *Poverty, Social Assistance, and the Employability of Mothers*, 23.
22. See Bradshaw et al., *Policy and Employment of Lone Parents*.
23. Land, "The Family Wage."
24. See Castles, "Needs-Based Strategies"; and Ian Shirley, Peggy Koopman-Boyden, Ian Pool, and Susan St. John, "Family Change and Family Policy in New Zealand," in *Family Change and Family Policies in Great Britain, Canada, New Zealand, and the United States*, ed. Kamerman and Kahn, 207–304.
25. See Julie White, *Sisters and Solidarity: Women and Unions in Canada* (Toronto: Thompson Educational, 1993), 24.
26. In New Zealand, union membership declined from about 60 percent of the employed labor force in 1945 to about 20 percent in 1996.
27. See Susan Pedersen, *Family, Dependence, and the Origins of the Welfare State: Britain and France, 1914–1945* (Cambridge: Cambridge University Press, 1993); Gisela Kaplan, *The Meagre Harvest: The Australian Women's Movement, 1950–1990s* (Sydney: Allen and Unwin, 1996); Baker and Phipps, "Family Change and Family Policy"; and Bashevkin, *Women on the Defensive*.
28. See Jane Ursel, *Private Lives, Public Policy: One Hundred Years of State Intervention in the Family* (Toronto: Women's Press, 1992).
29. See Maureen Baker, "Advocacy, Political Alliances, and the Implementation of Family Policies," in *Child and Family Policy: Struggles, Strategies, and Options*, ed. Jane Pulkingham and Gordon Ternowetsky (Toronto: Fernwood, 1997), 158–71.
30. During the early 1980s, REAL Women, an antifeminist and antiabortion organization, lobbied unsuccessfully for payments for mothers at home, as did the feminist umbrella group known as the National Action Committee on the Status of Women during the early 1980s. Groups including the National Action Committee, Women's Legal Education and Action Fund, and the Canadian Child Care Advocacy Association lobbied and litigated more successfully for employment, pay equity, and child-care subsidies for working women.

31. Vicky Randall, "Feminism and Child Daycare," *Journal of Social Policy* 25 (1996): 485–505.
32. Sylvia Bashevkin, "From Tough Times to Better Times: Feminism, Public Policy, and New Labour Politics in Britain," *International Political Science Review* 21 (2000): 407–24.
33. Bashevkin, *Women on the Defensive*, 210.
34. Baker and Tippin, *Poverty, Social Assistance, and the Employability of Mothers*, 253.
35. Ibid., 187.
36. See Esping-Andersen, *The Three Worlds of Welfare Capitalism*.
37. See O'Connor et al., *States, Markets, Families*.
38. It is notable that in 2000, New Zealand had a woman prime minister and a woman opposition leader.
39. See Helga Marie Hernes, *Welfare State and Women Power: Essays in State Feminism* (Oslo: Norwegian Press, 1987); and Marilyn Waring, *Counting for Nothing: What Men Value and What Women Are Worth* (Wellington, New Zealand: Allen and Unwin, 1988).
40. See Baker, *Canadian Family Policies*; and Diane Sainsbury, *Gender, Equality, and Welfare States* (Cambridge: Cambridge University Press, 1996).
41. Ruth Lister, "Citizenship Endangered," in *Critical Social Policy*, ed. David Taylor (London: Sage, 1996), 168–74.

5.
Road-Testing the Third Way

Single Mothers and Welfare Reform during the Clinton, Chrétien, and Blair Years

Sylvia Bashevkin

Introduction

Three nominally left-of-center political executives assumed office in major Anglo-American systems beginning in the early 1990s. U.S. president Bill Clinton, first elected in 1992; Canadian prime minister Jean Chrétien, first elected in 1993; and British prime minister Tony Blair, first elected in 1997, each defeated conservative leaders in their respective countries. In place of the cozy triumvirate that prevailed during the Ronald Reagan, Brian Mulroney, and Margaret Thatcher years, when neoconservatives were in charge, a "Third Way" triumvirate emerged of Clinton, Chrétien, and Blair.

Just what was this Third Way? What consequences did the switch from right-of-center toward nominally left-of-center political executives hold for citizens living in North America and Britain? In particular, what did Third Way leadership mean for one of the most contentious subjects of public debate during the 1990s—namely, the fate of lone mothers on social assistance benefits? This chapter addresses each question in turn, offering in the process a preliminary road test of Third Way public policy. The purpose of the road test is to move away from strictly conjectural claims about making left-of-center values relevant to the contemporary period, in order to consider how the ideas fare when, as the popular saying goes, the rubber hits the road.

This discussion is framed around the following core argument:

Third Way leaders often pursued a rhetoric on welfare reform that sounded more balanced and more compassionate than that of their conservative predecessors. However, the policies of the Clinton, Chrétien, and Blair years could produce a far more radically *conservative* restructuring of welfare regimes than was undertaken by Reagan, Mulroney, or even Thatcher. This chapter highlights three striking features to date of Third Way welfare reform in the Anglo-American world: first, the move toward what I term "work-tested" social benefits; second, shifts in the direction of what is referred to as taxified or fiscalized social policy; and third, parallel with Leah F. Vosko's argument in chapter 7, a growing emphasis on notions of economic or market-tested citizenship, in effect compromising older concepts of an expansive social citizenship.[1]

To begin with the first question, How do we define the Third Way? It is a slippery concept, with different meanings to different observers, and could hardly be said to command an overwhelming hold on the imagination of the Anglo-American electorate.[2] Each Third Way leader considered in this chapter was first elected as a top political executive with the support of just over 40 percent of the voting public: President Clinton won a 43 percent vote share in 1992 (when George Bush and Ross Perot shared the other 57 percent). Prime Minister Chrétien's Liberals in Canada won a majority government with 41 percent of the federal vote in 1993 (when a total of five parties won seats in the House of Commons). Prime Minister Blair's New Labour in Britain won a landslide majority with only 43 percent of the popular vote in 1997.

At the level of ideas, Clinton, Chrétien, and Blair articulated a view that individuals, no matter how modest their origins, could succeed in an opportunity-filled society as long as they were dutiful, responsible, and ambitious. In this respect, all three leaders fashioned a path to power to the right of the historically center-left positions of their respective parties. Clinton, Chrétien, and Blair embraced notions of individual ambition, maintained that the state's key job was enhancing opportunities for individual success, and emphasized the importance of personal duty and responsibility—elements drawn from traditional liberal and conservative doctrines. Like new conservatives, these leaders tended to look negatively on interest group and social movement mobilization, seeing collective action of that variety as inherently less legitimate than the actions of achieving individuals.

Yet Clinton, Chrétien, and Blair also dismissed what they portrayed as the extreme antisocietal notions of their conservative predecessors—by insisting that they were more compassionate, more balanced, and less dog-eat-dog social Darwinist than Reagan, Mulroney, or certainly Thatcher. Third Way leaders claimed they drew on the best in liberal, conservative, and social democratic traditions, merging these strengths, while rejecting the excesses of either unfettered individualism or unwieldy statism. As President Clinton argued with respect to the United States in his 1996 text titled *Between Hope and History*, "America is about *both* individual liberty and community obligation."[3]

Given these important similarities, what variations distinguished these three welfare states from each other? According to Esping-Andersen's comparative typology, all of the Anglo-American countries can be categorized as liberal, meaning neither social democratic nor corporatist, and residual welfare states.[4] None had a national child-care program, for example, and each one elevated or privileged the role of the market above that of the state.

Of the three cases, however, the United States was arguably the most bare-bones or residual welfare state. It alone, for example, lacked a universal health-care system in the 1990s. As well, the United States was distinctive because it contained the most powerful social or so-called moral right, an interest of particular concern to American scholars of welfare reform, including Gwendolyn Mink (see chapter 6). Along a continuum that would measure shifts in the direction of work-tested benefits, taxified social policy, and an increasingly tenuous or compromised notion of social citizenship, therefore, the United States was probably the most "developed" or "advanced" of these cases.

By way of comparison, Canada had a somewhat more robust welfare state than that of the United States. It offered universal health-care provisions during the 1990s, although the standards of the Canadian welfare state were widely viewed as in decline over time.[5] The social right in Canada was less influential than in the United States—meaning welfare debates at the federal level in Canada tended to focus less on such issues as teenage pregnancy and abortion than they did in the United States. Contemporary political developments in Canada, however, included the introduction of U.S.-style workfare provisions at the provincial level, as documented by Leah F. Vosko in chapter 7, as well as the rise of a strong social conservative presence in the leading federal opposition party, the Reform or Canadian Alliance organization.

Within this three-case comparison, the British welfare state was probably the most robust and the least influenced by social right interests. In the United Kingdom, as Maureen Baker shows in chapter 4, a less workerist view prevailed than in North America about what a "responsible" single parent—generally, a mother—should do while her children were young. American and Canadian policy makers tended to view mothers of very young children as employable in the thirty-plus hours of work per week category, while their British counterparts maintained that in the absence of decent child-care programs and fulfilling jobs, it might be preferable for the state to continue to pay social benefits to lone mothers with preschool children instead of pushing them into paid work.[6] With reference to notions of work-tested benefits, taxified social policy, and an eroded concept of social citizenship, the United Kingdom appeared to be less "advanced" or "developed" than Canada or certainly the United States.

Expectations of the Third Way

In what political context were Third Way leaders first elected? In *Women on the Defensive: Living through Conservative Times*, I traced the efforts of Margaret Thatcher, Ronald Reagan, Brian Mulroney, and their party successors to impose an individualist outlook that rejected the more collectivist ideas of their Labour, Democratic, and Liberal predecessors, as well as the organic community traditions of their own political parties.[7] Among the most concerted opponents of new conservative leaders were antipoverty and women's groups, which directed much of their criticism toward social assistance changes of the 1980s and following.

These changes included, in the United States, the 1988 Family Support Act, intended "to move single mothers off welfare through a combination of job training, work requirements, childcare subsidies, and child-support enforcement."[8] In Canada, the Mulroney government introduced what became known as the "cap on CAP," a decision that lowered federal social spending by placing a ceiling or cap on transfers via the Canada Assistance Plan (CAP) to the three wealthiest provinces to fund health, education, and welfare programs. This decision reduced federal transfers to Ontario, British Columbia, and Alberta by more than $2.1 billion between 1990 and 1995.[9] In Britain, Conservatives introduced the 1991 Child Support Act, which compelled single mothers on income support to name their child's father so that the Child Support Agency could obtain support payments from him and reduce welfare payments to her accordingly.[10]

Although the specific terms of these three conservative actions were far from identical, they contained important common threads and provoked somewhat similar opposition. What did social welfare interests in the United States, Canada, and Britain criticize about Republican and Tory social policy, and what, by way of implication, did they hope to see in the policies of "post-conservative" leaders? Five general criticisms stand out. First, conservative social policy focused on drawing public funds out of what were already modest, residual, and heavily means-tested income support programs. In Anglo-American systems, according to critics, introducing rigid work requirements, reducing federal social transfers to lower levels of government, and enforcing child-support payments all represented circuitous means used by conservative political executives to cut already limited welfare payments.

Second, progressives alleged that conservative rhetoric, especially in the United States and the United Kingdom, turned poverty from an economic condition into a cultural and—above all—a moral malady. The early manifestations of this approach in an American context are elucidated in Dionne Bensonsmith's work on the Moynihan Report, summarized in chapter 2 of this volume. The so-called family values discourse effectively defined single mothers trying to raise their children as "irresponsible" deviants who deserved public humiliation and other forms of state-sanctioned punishment. In the view of critics, negative talk about "dependence" and "irresponsibility" obscured the interconnectedness and what Selma Sevenhuijsen describes in chapter 1 as the interdependency that remain central to a healthy society; moreover, it neglected the fact that women's reliance on state benefits was in many cases preferable to their reliance on traditional forms of family organization.

Third, according to feminist and antipoverty interests, conservative efforts to push poor women, often from minority and immigrant backgrounds, into paid work ignored very significant patterns of sex segregation and pay differentials in the labor market. Welfare-to-work programs were unlikely to produce poverty-to-prosperity transformation for the simple reason that most single mothers "cannot get jobs that pay better than welfare."[11] Fourth, as argued by Gwendolyn Mink in chapter 6 and Leah F. Vosko in chapter 7 of this volume, pushing single mothers of young children into twenty or thirty or more hours of paid work per week denied the value of their unpaid child care and nurturing responsibilities and ignored the fact that public and workplace child-care programs were extremely limited in all of these countries. Finally, in North America, the decentralist impulse behind Reagan- and Mulroney-era actions was seen as threatening to accelerate a "race to the bottom" in these federal systems, where social assistance was already based on localized "patchworks" comprised of individual state and provincial schemes.[12] Further decentralization, according to observers on the left, risked undermining the already fragile idea of national social standards in federal systems.

To the extent that progressive critics of conservative social policy prescribed core goals for "post-conservative" leaders, these tended to include: (1) ending cuts to already threadbare income support programs; (2) resisting the use of punitive, moralistic discourse about welfare and single motherhood; (3) paying attention to labor market issues of sex segregation and unequal pay in designing training, apprenticeship, and work programs; (4) creating high-quality, affordable, and universal child-care programs; and (5) in federal systems, refusing to grant greater leverage to subnational levels of government.

It seems fair to suggest that Third Way leaders elected to office in these three countries since 1992 have *not*—at least, not yet—fulfilled these expectations. What they have done, however, is to raise and subsequently dampen the expectations of many progressive experts, as well as campaigners. We can examine the evidence to date, case by case.

The American Case

If we begin with the United States in the period 1992 through 2000, we recall in President Clinton a political executive with overpowering personal drive, boundless ambition, and an unwavering belief in the capacity of motivated individuals to overcome huge obstacles. The campaign rhetoric of candidate Clinton in 1992 emphasized "ending welfare as we know it," making welfare "a second chance and not a way of life," and focusing on "the economy, stupid," so that enterprising individuals could grasp the gold ring called the American Dream. Clinton promised to "make work pay," in his words, by first, expanding tax incentives under the Earned Income Tax Credit (EITC) for low-income parents to pursue paid employment instead of welfare, and second, raising the level of the U.S. national minimum wage.[13] Raising the EITC was consistent with arguments in many Anglo-American systems about the need to help poor working families who did not receive various benefits that *were* available to welfare recipients.

It is certainly plausible to argue that candidate Clinton's expansive ideas about education, job training, health care, and other issues were stopped in their tracks by a re-energized Republican right. Especially following the switch from Democratic to Republican control in both houses of Congress in 1994, Bill Clinton was forced to deal with a far less congenial legislative branch of government. Yet Clinton's own ideas about social welfare in particular were from the outset those of a pragmatic, small-state governor, one who wanted to see a further shift of authority away from federal and toward state and local levels of government.[14]

The welfare reform proposals put forward by the Clinton White House before Republicans won control on Capitol Hill in 1994 were conservative and decentralist, relative to where most U.S. Democrats had stood in the past. The Clinton plan permitted states to impose child-exclusion rules, meaning higher benefits could be denied for children born or conceived while the mother was on the existing system of social assistance in the United States, known as Aid to Families with Dependent Children (AFDC). This focus on giving the states more power over welfare was consistent with Clinton's prior record as president (and the record of his predecessor in the White House, George Bush) of giving waivers to states to allow them to undertake a variety of social assistance "experiments" that would form a "laboratory" for national policy changes. Furthermore, Clinton's plan offered some help with child-care expenses for the working poor, as an incentive to keep single mothers in particular off welfare; it suggested a very gradual phase-in of work requirements so that about 10 percent of adults in AFDC households would be in government or government-subsidized jobs within six years (by 2000). In order to pay for work subsidies, child-care subsidies, and so on, Bill Clinton's plan reduced welfare benefits for noncitizens (including legal immigrants) and for people disabled due to drug or alcohol abuse.[15]

The welfare reform bill ultimately signed by President Clinton in 1996 bore a much closer resemblance to Republican proposals coming out of the 1994 Contract with America than to his own earlier positions—although it must be emphasized that Clinton's own proposals were focused on cutting welfare spending and pressing the work option. The 1996 Personal Responsibility and Work Opportunity Reconciliation Act (PRWORA) eliminated the AFDC program and replaced it with a new block grant scheme called Temporary Assistance for Needy Families. The bill reduced federal government spending on welfare by about $55 billion over six years.[16] It imposed "hard time limits," meaning adults could receive welfare benefits to a lifetime maximum of five years, but less if states so decide. States had six years as of 1996 to ensure that 50 percent of their welfare recipients were in work activities. According to the terms of the bill, half of all single parents on welfare would be expected to work thirty hours per week within six years.[17]

Of particular interest to feminist analysts were the components of PRWORA that dealt with paternity and out-of-marriage births. Under the terms of PRWORA, all welfare mothers must disclose the paternity of their children; teenage mothers have to live with their parents or other adults and participate in education or training programs to be eligible for assistance. Moreover, states that successfully reduced out-of-wedlock births without increasing abortion rates became eligible under the 1996 legislation for extra federal funds under the terms of an "illegitimacy bonus." States were offered the right to impose child exclusion rules or "family caps," meaning that higher benefits could be denied for children born or conceived by a mother on cash assistance. Overall, the 1996 legislation eliminated any legally enforceable right of individuals to collect social assistance and introduced provisions that, in the words of Gwendolyn Mink, "pressure poor single mothers to surrender their civil rights as a condition of economic assistance."[18]

Proponents of U.S. welfare reform were quick to argue that the 1996 bill went a long way toward "ending welfare as we know it." President Clinton and others frequently pointed to very low rates of unemployment in the United States, declining welfare case loads, and sustained job growth. Yet a more analytic look at the same scenario suggested that work requirements in the United States tended to push better-educated, better-skilled, and less "difficult" social assistance recipients into paid employment, while at the same time leaving those with more limited skills dependent on shrinking and time-limited welfare benefits.[19] Would the paid work found by former welfare recipients in the United States provide a survivable wage? Would it displace other women and men in better-paid, unionized public service jobs and thus accelerate a state-by-state "race to the bottom" of social standards? How quickly and dramatically would an economic recession in the United States overturn the pattern of declining welfare case loads? What might happen to state-level welfare programs once the front-ended federal money promised in 1996 began to dry up? These remain important questions open to speculation, and difficult to research, largely because "most [U.S.] states do not have the capacity to effectively trace ... families [who have left the welfare rolls], even to find out if they have remained employed."[20]

Given the harsh criticism he faced from some quarters, how was President Clinton able to sign this bill? One explanation draws on Paul Pierson's theory of welfare state retrenchment, which says that leaders manage to contract or shrink state programs when there is credit to be claimed and blame to be avoided.[21] In the case of PRWORA, Clinton could claim policy credit for reducing spending and "fixing" welfare by rewarding work, at the same time that he could avoid blame by shifting already devolved program responsibility to state governments. Second, following the lines of feminist claims about the unequal consequences of both welfare state expansion and contraction, it can be argued that eliminating AFDC as a federal entitlement program and replacing it with a more residual, decentralized, and socially invasive regime essentially placed the human burden of welfare reform on a less-than-crucial political constituency for Bill Clinton—namely, impoverished single mother–led households, more than half of them with minority backgrounds in the 1990s.[22]

The move toward a taxified or fiscalized social policy in the United States is reflected in the growing size of the Earned Income Tax Credit. During his first term in office, President Clinton won an increase in the EITC that constituted less than three-quarters of what he had promised during the 1992 election campaign. Even so, by 1996, federal spending on the EITC reached nearly $25 billion, or nearly twice as much as the federal government had been spending on the old AFDC program.[23] Because an enriched Earned Income Tax Credit corresponded closely with public pressures to reward work instead of welfare, Republicans in Congress were less effective in their efforts to derail Clinton on this issue than they were in other areas—notably, health-care reform.

In short, the Clinton legacy included heavy rhetorical emphasis on "the work alternative" to welfare, as well as policy shifts toward a higher minimum wage and tax subsidies for low-income workers under the EITC. One can thus identify three discernible shifts in Clinton-era social policy: first, a move in the direction of "work-testing" what were already residual, means-tested social benefits; second, a shift toward taxifying and individualizing social policy such that it was taken out of the realm of direct legislative expenditure and, in many respects, removed from explicit public debate (the obvious example here was the enriched Earned Income Tax Credit); and third, a trend toward equating labor market participation with citizenship, such that the older right to public assistance based on need was replaced by a notion of temporary assistance only, based on paid labor force engagement. In this manner, citizenship no longer resonated with T. H. Marshall's concept of a broad spectrum of social rights and engagements available to all,[24] because citizenship became economically contingent, based on paid employment only, which in turn tended to be more tenuous, short term, and nonunionized over time. As Selma Sevenhuijsen's and Jane Jenson's discussions in this volume suggest, people who were unpaid caregivers and others who did not work for pay thus began to reside outside the boundaries of a highly compromised version of American social citizenship.

The Canadian Case

If we turn to the case of Prime Minister Chrétien, we find a Canadian leader described by his biographer as a "great master of the middle" in the tradition of another very successful federal Liberal politician, Mackenzie King.[25] Commitment to the values of personal drive, discipline, and hard work were vividly embodied in Chrétien's own life experience. According to journalist Lawrence Martin, these core norms underpinned Jean Chrétien's elevation of practical action above ideas in politics. Known as a tornado by those who have worked with him,[26] Chrétien consistently rejected what he referred to in his own memoirs as "doctrinaire" solutions to problems.[27] In *Straight from the Heart*, first published in 1985, Chrétien wrote with great enthusiasm about the fruits of private sector investment in Canada and, with equal fervor, about the good things government has done for Canadians.[28] Like other Third Way leaders, Chrétien rejected what Anthony Giddens referred to as the "market fundamentalism" of conservatives,[29] at the same time as he was impatient with the narrowly statist solutions of the political left—and particularly impatient with what Chrétien described in 1985 as the "idle hands and lost pride" caused by a social safety net that "undermines incentive and is abused."[30]

This same basic outlook was presented in the Liberal Red Book, the party's electoral platform for the 1993 federal campaign. General statements about the Liberal commitment to "fundamental fairness and dignity" and a pooling of social resources in the wake of what were presented as destructive Conservative policies appeared alongside arguments that older forms of passive social assistance created dependence and disincentives to work.[31] Individuals, according to the Red Book, need to become self-sufficient by working, thus moving "from dependence to full participation in the economic and social life of Canada."[32] In particular, single mothers on welfare can "break the chain of dependence" once a more expansive national child-care system was set in place through joint federal/provincial efforts.[33] Yet as of late 2001, during Chrétien's third term as leader of a majority Liberal government, no national child-care system had arrived on Canadian earth. Moreover, federal Liberals during the Chrétien years embarked on a process of deficit-fighting plus social policy decentralization and retrenchment that vastly eclipsed anything pursued by capital-C Conservatives during the Mulroney years.

What are the consequences thus far of social policy change during the Chrétien years? Eliminating the cost-shared Canada Assistance Plan and replacing it with the block-funded Canada Health and Social Transfer (CHST), as announced in the 1995 federal budget, entailed multibillion-dollar cuts in federal transfers to the provinces and involved major reductions in federal controls over how provinces spend money—with virtually no conditions attached, for example, to how much funds subnational governments devote to health versus postsecondary education versus social assistance. As announced by Finance Minister Paul Martin, the CHST reduced federal grants to the provinces by more than $7 billion during its first two years of operation. This constituted about a 40-percent reduction in federal social transfers to the provinces.[34] Observers portrayed the change from an open-ended cost-sharing framework between the federal and provincial governments under the 1966 Canada Assistance Plan to the close-ended block transfer under the CHST, beginning in 1996, as evidence that deficit reduction had become the top priority of the federal cabinet. According to one account, introducing the CHST allowed the Finance Department in Canada "to impose its own unilateral fiscal fix on the country's social programs."[35]

Above all, with respect to social citizenship, ending the Canada Assistance Plan extinguished crucial guidelines in place since 1966 to the effect that persons in need had the right to income support and the right to appeal denial of that support through a provincially established appeals process. Although the 1966 Canada Assistance Plan "prohibited the provinces from requiring social assistance applicants to accept employment *as a condition of receiving assistance,"*[36] the CHST contained no such provision. As Leah F. Vosko demonstrates in chapter 7, eliminating the no-workfare guideline at the federal level as of 1996 left the door open for provincial governments to introduce schemes like Ontario Works.

In quantitative terms, data show that Canadian provinces as a group spent less per person on social assistance after 1995 than before, with Ontario and Alberta leading the way on cuts to welfare rates and tightened eligibility rules.[37] As well, the gap between the after-tax income of rich and poor in Canada widened after the federal Liberals came to power in 1993, largely because of spending reductions in the areas of social assistance and unemployment insurance. In particular, data released by the federally funded National Council of Welfare showed an increase after 1995—the year the CHST was announced—in the already high percentage of young, single mother led families living in poverty—from 83 percent in 1995 to more than 91 percent in subsequent years.[38] Various measures of child poverty in Canada also showed higher absolute numbers and higher relative percentages over time—and once again, the most common explanation was reduced federal transfers and reduced federal controls on provincial action under the CHST, along with major federal cuts to unemployment insurance and significant provincial cuts to social assistance programs.

In short, Canada was governed after 1993 by a pragmatic prime minister from modest origins who believed hard-working people like himself could succeed despite the odds. Together with Finance Minister Paul Martin, Jean Chrétien moved the federal budget from serious deficit to considerable surplus—but at the not insignificant cost of lowered federal transfers to the provinces, vastly weakened federal control over those reduced transfers, an increasingly wide gap between haves and have-nots in Canadian society, and, in national terms, an extinguishment of crucial social citizenship principles dating from 1966.

How did Prime Minister Chrétien manage to make these changes? Like President Clinton, his success was contingent on an ingenious combination of claiming credit and avoiding blame. Creating the CHST allowed federal Liberals to argue that they were taking seriously the need to control spending, reduce the deficit, and encourage policy flexibility in a diverse federation. Like the Clinton Democrats, the Chrétien Liberals could claim that their actions responded to public concerns about overly generous social assistance programs.[39] Moreover, again like their American counterparts, Canadian Liberals could hope to escape responsibility for the negative fallout from these changes by using the complex terms of federal/provincial fiscal relations as a convenient cover.

This retrenchment argument needs to be refined, however, by reference to feminist theories of unequal consequence. The CHST eliminated what had been an open-ended federal cost-sharing arrangement under CAP to pay half of provincial and territorial social assistance and social service expenditures. Roughly 70 percent of single parents in Canada, most of them women, received some form of social assistance in the 1990s. Moreover, social service funding under CAP included subsidies for low-income child care and shelters for battered women.[40] The reduction in funds going to the provinces under the CHST, together with an end to the older CAP principles that persons in need had the right to income and could appeal welfare decisions, revealed a clear fiscal and jurisdictional retreat by the federal government from an area of critical importance to poor women.[41]

As well, the vast bulk of Canadian welfare state workers in the education, health-care, and social service fields were female and, compared with the United States, they were more likely to be unionized public sector employees.[42] Canadian women therefore faced very specific risks under the CHST, both as welfare state clients and as workers, even though the terms of the Transfer contained none of the socially invasive regulations about paternity, illegitimacy, and teenage motherhood that were found in American reforms of the same period (for more on these provisions, see part IV of this volume). Like Bill Clinton, Jean Chrétien was hardly punished in electoral terms for his decision to restructure federal social assistance arrangements.

The changeover from CAP to the CHST in Canada was

accompanied by the introduction of a National Child Benefit, under which universal family allowances were replaced by a new benefit payable primarily to low-income employed parents through the tax system. As of 2001, the National Child Benefit was not passed on to parents on welfare in eight out of the ten Canadian provinces. The two provinces where it was transferred to parents on welfare, New Brunswick and Newfoundland, contained only about 5 percent of the national population. Supporters claimed that the National Child Benefit offered a worthy, targeted approach to assisting low-income families.[43] Critics portrayed it as little more than "a work-incentive program" that reinforced the efforts of some relatively wealthy and populous Canadian provinces (notably, Ontario and Alberta) to emulate U.S.-style workfare programs.[44] Even its most fervent admirers admitted that the National Child Benefit was at best a small first step toward reforming social policy in Canada. With a projected cost of $1.7 billion in the year 2000, it was expected to assist only about 12 percent of low-income, single-parent families.[45]

Overall, the evidence to date suggested Canadian social policy during the Chrétien years moved in the direction of work-tested social benefits, particularly with the end of a no-work-for-welfare provision under the CHST in 1996; an increasingly taxified or fiscalized social policy, with the National Child Benefit as Canada's latest targeted program for low-income families; and an assumption that active labor force participation was the sine qua non of contemporary citizenship. As Margaret Little argued in her account of welfare reform in Canada, eliminating universal family allowances meant that governments at all levels could focus their attention on "worthy" workers eligible for new, narrowly targeted programs like the National Child Benefit. In Little's words, "the demise of universal family allowances further impoverished unemployable single mothers in relation to the working poor. Through the child tax benefit single mothers were financially penalized if they were not involved in paid work."[46]

The British Case

Turning to the final case of Third Way leadership under examination, that of Prime Minister Tony Blair, it is important to emphasize that Britain remains a unitary state. Although New Labour pursued a devolution scheme that granted increased parliamentary autonomy to Scotland and Wales and greater authority to local governments, the plan was not to create a decentralized social policy arrangement comparable to those of either the United States or Canada in the 1990s. Moreover, unlike the United States during the Clinton years and Canada during the Chrétien era, Britain under Tony Blair was committed to spending more, rather than less, money on its welfare reform project. The New Deal, a welfare-to-work scheme announced by Labour while it was still in opposition, would be financed by about £5.2 billion in new windfall profits tax money.[47] This fiscal infusion meant that New Labour's approach diverged from the budget reduction or retrenchment rationale that rested behind North American decisions to eliminate the AFDC program, as well as the Canada Assistance Plan.

How did Tony Blair frame discussions of work and welfare? First of all, Blair, like Clinton, spoke at length about education—meaning higher standards in state schools, the creation of more community college–type options for the middle third of the educational ladder, and lots of training (mostly provided by employers) for people reliant on social benefits. Second, he stressed the need to build in Britain a society with greater opportunities, "where everyone has a stake" and where "ambition is matched by compassion, success by social justice, and rewards by responsibility."[48] Blair's notion of a stakeholder economy was grounded in his view of a wealth-creating (rather than the Old Labour emphasis on a wealth-distributing) system, "in which opportunity is extended, merit rewarded and no group of individuals locked out."[49] Excluded people, defined as those without paid employment who often lived in "workless households," were the target population for a new government bureau called the Social Exclusion Unit.

Critics argued that despite this talk about social inclusion, the New Labour project for welfare reform was in fact quite exclusionary, since it refused to acknowledge that people could be part of society if they were not working for pay. Commentators frequently cited a 1997 statement by New Labour's first minister for social security, Harriet Harman, to the effect that "Life is about work, not just about claiming benefits."⁵⁰ The decisions of the Blair government to cut single-parent benefit premiums in 1997 and disability benefits in 1999 reinforced critics' contentions that a narrow, punitive, and work-obsessed rationale loomed large in New Labour social policy.

The parameters of this record are still emerging, since New Labour remained at this writing at the start of its second government mandate, after winning the June 2001 elections. Yet the broad lines of a Tony Blair Third Way on social policy can be discerned. To date, the New Deal on welfare-to-work has focused primarily on improving the employability of 18- to 24-year-olds. Officially unemployed youth who had not worked for at least six months were offered a four-month "Gateway period" that provided job counseling and advice. After four months, they would select one of four options: subsidized jobs, full-time education or training, voluntary sector work, or environmental work. As New Labour politicians consistently emphasized, "there is no fifth option."

The Blair government introduced far smaller New Deal programs for single parents and disabled people, in which participation was not initially compulsory. They also brought in a Working Families Tax Credit, modeled on the Earned Income Tax Credit in the United States, along with a national minimum wage. Taken as a group, these New Labour provisions were generally viewed by social welfare interests as useful, although quite limited, first steps in the direction of assisting people—many of them women—in low-wage work.

What can be said about Blair government decisions thus far? First, social policy changes bore a striking resemblance to earlier actions in North America, in the sense of emphasizing incentives for people to get off welfare and work for pay. The New Deal for the young unemployed was in this sense a work-tested social benefit, although it was also education-tested in the sense that high school vocational training was nationally subsidized. Second, like its Third Way counterparts in the United States and Canada, New Labour pursued social policy initiatives using labor market and tax vehicles, rather than traditional spending programs. Relevant examples of this shift included the creation of a national minimum wage, as well as the Working Families Tax Credit.

However, some Labour government directions had a distinctly

British twist. Welfare to work in the United Kingdom, for example, explicitly permitted the unionization of New Deal workers and established a minimum wage for New Deal workers. This was not the case throughout the United States or, for that matter, in some Canadian provinces, including Ontario. As well, the fact that participation in New Deal welfare-to-work programs was not initially compulsory for single parents and the disabled meant that British notions of citizenship were not entirely commodified, or transformed from expansive social notions to solely economic and labor market ones. In Britain, therefore, there existed some official recognition during New Labour's first term in office that people could participate in and contribute to society other than through paid work. Worries were voiced, however, that the limited uptake of paid work by lone parents in Britain would lead to more punitive policies under a second Blair government. As of April 2001, for example, new claimants for Income Support benefits in Britain faced a compulsory work-focused interview as part of the benefits application process, as long as their youngest child was five years of age or older.

Drawing Conclusions

It is instructive to step back from the empirical details to look for evidence of cross-national convergence and divergence. In terms of spillover across Anglo-American boundaries, we can see clear evidence on both sides of the 49th parallel of further policy decentralization, a shared move toward block-grant funding, and a common erosion of social citizenship norms. In the United States and Canada, Clinton- and Chrétien-era decisions replaced shared-cost federal social programs with block grants (or fixed, lump-sum payments), cut spending on cash benefits, awarded greater control over social policy to subnational governments, and stripped what remained of a national entitlement to income support based on need. This record eclipsed in a regressive way not only Republican and Conservative precedents in this field, but also Democratic and Liberal campaign promises.

The extent to which North American welfare policy at the federal level moved in restrictive directions following 1993, however, varied quite a bit. Provisions of the U.S. Personal Responsibility and Work Opportunity Reconciliation Act ended the AFDC program, imposed time limits and work requirements for benefits, insisted that all mothers applying for social assistance disclose the paternity of their children, and offered financial bonuses to states that reduced nonmarital births, but kept abortion rates from rising. The Canada Health and Social Transfer eliminated what had been an open-ended cost-sharing deal for provincial and territorial social assistance and social service programs, but contained none of the socially invasive regulations about paternity or illegitimacy that were present in U.S. reforms of the same period. Since the Transfer did not prohibit the introduction of such provisions by provinces, some subnational governments (including in wealthy jurisdictions such as Ontario, discussed in chapter 7 by Leah F. Vosko) moved directly into the breach that opened up in 1996.

In Britain, the Blair government instituted a voluntary job counseling, training, and placement program for single parents, during the same term as it carried out a very controversial Tory promise to scrap lone-parent premiums for social benefits. Overall, New Labour's directions in office were more consistent with the expectations of a Third Way government than were those of Democratic and Liberal political executives in the United States and Canada. Yet Tony Blair's campaign talk about rebuilding frayed fabrics and promoting social inclusion gave way over time to far less tolerant language that sounded more like that of his Tory predecessors and of U.S. politicians. Prime Minister Blair spoke in 1998, for example, of ending "the something-for-nothing welfare state."[51] Given the heightened emphasis of Blair and his acolytes on notions of personal duty and responsibility, these statements suggested that during a second term in office, Labour might be willing to adopt the more punitive directions of North American welfare reform initiatives. In other words, continued diffusion across the Atlantic seemed likely under a second New Labour government.

The main bits of evidence for cross-national similarity, then, were as follows. First, beleaguered social citizenship norms in each of these countries came under sustained siege during the mid-1990s and following. The idea of a fulsome right to social engagement, available to all regardless of sex, economic status, race, family status, or other factors, was clearly endangered by the highly invasive terms of PRWORA, signed in the summer of 1996 by President Clinton. Decisions in Canada to eliminate most federal guidelines for social programs (except in the field of health care) as of 1996 opened the way for provinces to adopt elements of U.S. welfare reform policy, including socially conservative, "family values" regulations, along with compulsory work for welfare. As well, changes to the social assistance appeals process in all three countries, including Britain under New Labour, directly undermined any assumption of a latent right to benefits.[52]

Second, Third Way leaders tended to prioritize pro-market, paid-work-is-all-that-matters principles. Each introduced or, in the U.S. case, enriched a system of tax-based employment incentives—termed work-tested benefits—that differed from traditional social spending programs. The expansion of the Earned Income Tax Credit under the Clinton administration, the creation of a National Child Benefit in Canada during the Chrétien years, and the introduction of a Working Families Tax Credit by New Labour in Britain all reflected growing reliance on complex fiscal maneuvers to "fix" social problems. Operating in the arcane domain of economists and tax specialists, rather than in the more accessible world of social workers and antipoverty activists, these provisions tended to address welfare in a manner that moved questions about human needs from the remit of social service and labor departments to the purview of finance or treasury departments. A technical discourse about tax incentives to foster paid employment thus overshadowed older concerns about food, shelter, basic income, and labor market regulations, as a fiscalized and work-tested outlook came to dominate Anglo-American social policy debates.

In short, core shared elements of the Third Way record rested in the promotion of not only a tenuous and compromised form of social citizenship, but also a work-tested, increasingly fiscalized view of social policy. At the level of explanation, these patterns can be linked to a pragmatic recognition by Clinton, Chrétien, and Blair that it was easier to run with than oppose the prevailing moralistic climate of opinion on welfare reform. Hiding new social expenditures in tax-based programs for working adults provided a convenient alternative to higher-visibility spending schemes that rested outside the tax regime. Moreover, particularly in the United States and Canada, fiscal and decentralist pressures from an energized political right meant that these were "post-conservative" times in name only. Both Bill Clinton and Jean Chrétien appropriated conservative language and arguments in their efforts to claim credit for lowering welfare spending and, at the same time, increasing the flexibility available to subnational governments in federal systems.

A number of larger questions follow from these comparative conclusions. First of all, will Third Way changes in terms of work-testing social benefits, taxifying social policy, and placing constraints on older, more expansive concepts of social citizenship do much about poverty as we know it? This line of inquiry overlooks a fundamental point: that is, once poverty was defined as a moral problem, rather than as an economic or social issue, as occurred clearly in the United States and to some extent in Canada and Britain as well, it made a huge difference whether people were poor while working versus poor while on benefits. To proponents of an unwavering pro-work, anti-"dependence," and pro–"personal responsibility" approach, the pursuit of punitive solutions became not just morally defensible, but also ethically essential. At its core, the "moral right" argument about poverty said that it didn't matter if people had enough to eat—they just needed the proper values about work.

Second, how did public policy reach this point? A broader argument with respect to the erosion of social citizenship can be stated as follows: From an emphasis through the interwar and postwar decades on collective and especially state responsibility for society's less fortunate members, the climate of ideas moved over time, even on the political center and center-left, toward an increasingly individualistic stress on notions of personal responsibility. Responsible citizens, in the jargon of the Third Way, were those who took care of themselves and those around them, meaning that they were not dependent on state transfers. If they were allowed to be state-dependent for a temporary period of time, then it was only with the proviso that they were actively seeking work and actively making themselves more work-ready.

In reviewing three contemporary Third Way leaders, this discussion points to their shared emphasis on the responsibility of individuals to take up the opportunities that market economies offer. According to Bill Clinton, Jean Chrétien, and Tony Blair, people from modest social origins can succeed despite the odds. They just need—in the words of Clinton and Blair—"a hand up, not a hand out." The role of the state from this perspective is to act as a facilitator, both for dutiful, "moral" action on the part of individuals and for "responsible" investments on the part of private employers. Using labor market, social policy, and taxation levers, the state presses individuals to work, just as it uses low taxes and constrained social benefits to encourage businesses to locate in a given jurisdiction. The fact that in federal systems like those of the United States and Canada, the national government ceded a great deal more authority to subnational levels during the Clinton and Chrétien years—especially in an area like social assistance policy, where subnational units long wielded considerable clout—meant that federal governments were becoming primarily rhetorical facilitators of what appeared to be an increasingly moralistic agenda about personal responsibility. In short, unlike the situation during the Lyndon Johnson or Pierre Trudeau years in North America, when national elites invested money, as well as rhetoric, behind a socioeconomic "war on poverty," one could argue that their Third Way counterparts withdrew funds and put a renewed rhetorical push behind a moralistic "war against poor people."

What about people who were not "responsible," in the jargon of the Third Way? Was this just another way of returning to older notions of the deserving versus the undeserving poor—with the virtuous widow epitomizing the deserving social assistance recipient, for example, and the unmarried teenage mother as the undeserving one? One could argue that there was nothing new about regulating and categorizing the poor, that we simply saw new jargon in the 1990s for setting up the terms of the very old "moral" debate about good versus evil.

Perhaps some new angles did emerge to shape the contemporary debate. First of all, there existed a fundamental tension in Third

Way discourse between the emphasis on personal independence, on the one hand, and a new communitarian focus on healthy societies, on the other. It seemed difficult for leaders like Clinton, Chrétien, and Blair to claim with much credibility that they were societally conscious when they pushed so hard on ideas of personal responsibility and independence that citizens heard very, very little about notions of interdependence—except when it had to do with the nuclear, and predominantly heterosexual, family unit. Given the economic insecurity and profound anxiety of these times, was there not something to be said for human interdependence on a larger scale?

Second, it seemed that Third Way ideas and policies about welfare reform contained a fundamentally authoritarian streak. As Ralf Dahrendorf remarked in an article in *Foreign Affairs*, there was something unsettling about leaders who said that the state "will no longer pay for things but will tell people what to do."[53] Dahrendorf claimed that Clinton, Blair, and company tossed aside fundamental notions of human liberty in their pursuit of social cohesion—but one could go further and ask if indeed social cohesion was any more central to the Third Way world view than was individual liberty. Ralf Dahrendorf's questions about the Third Way in Britain were particularly important because they reinforced many similar concerns raised by welfare reform critics in Canada and the United States.

This road test of the Third Way public policies of Clinton, Chrétien, and Blair in the area of social assistance suggests that welfare reform under their watch may turn out to be substantially more radical *in a conservative direction* than either their rhetoric may have indicated or their conservative predecessors managed to accomplish. The shifts underway since the early 1990s appear to be significant and, as social scientists, it's *our* job—or, in the jargon of the Third Way, our duty and responsibility—to subject these actions to very close scrutiny.

Notes

Research for this study was supported by the Social Sciences and Humanities Research Council of Canada. All monetary amounts in the text are cited in the currency of the country in question.

1. For a discussion of marketized and individualized citizenship patterns with reference to one case, see Jane Jenson and Susan D. Phillips, "Regime Shift: New Citizenship Practices in Canada," *International Journal of Canadian Studies* 14 (1996): 111–35.
2. For a comparative exploration of these themes, see Donley T. Studlar, "The Politics of the Third Way: Highway to the Future or Political Parking Lot," paper prepared for "Between Integration and Disintegration" conference at the University of Oklahoma, February 2000.
3. President Bill Clinton, *Between Hope and History: Meeting America's Challenges for the 21st Century* (New York: Random House, 1996), 117. Emphasis in original.
4. See Gøsta Esping-Andersen, *Politics against Markets: The Social Democratic Road to Power* (Princeton: Princeton University Press, 1985); and Gøsta Esping-Andersen, *The Three Worlds of Welfare Capitalism* (Princeton: Princeton University Press, 1990).
5. See, for example, Raymond B. Blake, Penny E. Bryden, and J. Frank Strain, eds., *The Welfare State in Canada: Past, Present and Future* (Toronto: Irwin, 1997).
6. For comparative treatments of this debate, see Maureen Baker and David Tippin, *Poverty, Social Assistance, and the Employability of Mothers: Restructuring Welfare States* (Toronto: University of Toronto Press, 1999); and Julia O'Connor, Ann Shola Orloff, and Sheila Shaver, *States, Markets, Families: Gender, Liberalism, and Social Policy in Australia, Canada, Great Britain and the United States* (Cambridge: Cambridge University Press, 1999).
7. Sylvia Bashevkin, *Women on the Defensive: Living through Conservative Times* (Chicago: University of Chicago Press, 1998).
8. Kathryn Edin and Christopher Jencks, "Welfare," in Christopher Jencks, *Rethinking Social Policy: Race, Poverty, and the Underclass* (Cambridge: Harvard University Press, 1992), 204.
9. Margaret Little, *"No Car, No Radio, No Liquor Permit": The Moral Regulation of Single Mothers in Ontario, 1920–1997* (Toronto: Oxford University Press, 1998), 151.
10. See Jane Millar, "State, Family, and Personal Responsibility: The Changing Balance for Lone Mothers in the UK," in *Women and Social Policy*, ed. Jo Campling, 2nd ed. (London: Macmillan, 1997), 154–62.
11. Edin and Jencks, "Welfare," 204.
12. See Gerard Boychuk, *Patchworks of Purpose: The Development of Provincial Social Assistance Regimes in Canada* (Montreal: McGill-Queen's University Press, 1998). In Canada, opposition to decentralization was strongest outside Quebec.
13. On Clinton's rhetoric and campaign promises, see R. Kent Weaver, "Ending Welfare as We Know It," in *The Social Divide: Political Parties and the Future of Activist Government*, ed. Margaret Weir (Washington, D.C.: Brookings Institution, 1998), 361–416.
14. See Clinton, *Between Hope and History*, 92.

15. See Gary Bryner, *Politics and Public Morality: The Great American Welfare Reform Debate* (New York: Norton, 1998), 76–86.
16. Boychuk, *Patchworks of Purpose*, 104.
17. See Bryner, *Politics and Public Morality*, 175–81.
18. Gwendolyn Mink, *Welfare's End* (Ithaca, N.Y.: Cornell University Press, 1998), 2.
19. See Demetra Smith Nightingale and Robert H. Haveman, eds., *The Work Alternative: Welfare Reform and the Realities of the Job Market* (Washington, D.C.: Urban Institute, 1995); and Joel F. Handler and Lucie White, eds., *Hard Labor: Women and Work in the Post-Welfare Era* (Armonk, N.Y.: M. E. Sharpe, 1999).
20. Weaver, "Ending Welfare as We Know It," 403.
21. Paul Pierson, *Dismantling the Welfare State? Reagan, Thatcher, and the Politics of Retrenchment* (Cambridge: Cambridge University Press, 1994).
22. For a critique of Pierson's account in light of feminist theorizing, see Sylvia Bashevkin, "Rethinking Retrenchment: North American Social Policy during the Early Clinton and Chrétien Years," *Canadian Journal of Political Science* 33 (2000): 7–36.
23. See Weaver, "Ending Welfare as We Know It," 398.
24. See T. H. Marshall, "Citizenship and Social Class," in T. H. Marshall and Tom Bottomore, *Citizenship and Social Class* (London: Pluto, 1992).
25. Lawrence Martin, *Chrétien, Volume 1: The Will to Win* (Toronto: Lester Publishing, 1995), 376.
26. Ibid., 236.
27. Jean Chrétien, *Straight from the Heart* (Toronto: Key Porter, 1985), 219.
28. See, for example, Chrétien's comments in his memoirs about the condition of his home town of Shawinigan, Quebec (ibid., 114).
29. Anthony Giddens, "Better Than Warmed-over Porridge," *New Statesman* (February 12, 1999), 25. See also Anthony Giddens, *The Third Way: The Renewal of Social Democracy* (Cambridge: Polity, 1998).
30. Chrétien, *Straight from the Heart*, 114.
31. *Creating Opportunity: The Liberal Plan for Canada* (Ottawa: Liberal Party of Canada, 1993), 73.
32. Ibid., 21.
33. Ibid., 39.
34. See Douglas Durst, "Phoenix or Fizzle? Background to Canada's New National Child Benefit," in *Canada's National Child Benefit*, ed. Douglas Durst (Halifax: Fernwood, 1999), 13.
35. Edward Greenspon and Anthony Wilson-Smith, *Double Vision: The Inside Story of the Liberals in Power* (Toronto: Doubleday, 1996), 230.
36. Allan Moscovitch, "The Canada Health and Social Transfer," in *The Welfare State in Canada*, Blake et al., 107. Emphasis in original.
37. One of the first actions of the Conservative government elected in

Ontario in 1995 was to cut welfare benefit rates by nearly 21 percent. See Bruce Little, "Welfare Has Endured the Biggest Cuts," *Globe and Mail*, January 11, 1999, B5.

38. Graham Fraser, "Poverty Rates Rising, Report Says," *Globe and Mail*, May 12, 1998, A4.
39. On the dynamics of public support for welfare programs in the United States, see Stephen M. Teles, *Whose Welfare? AFDC and Elite Politics* (Lawrence: University Press of Kansas, 1998), chap. 3; and R. Kent Weaver, "Ending Welfare as We Know It," 2000, chap. 7. Canadian data are presented in Alan Toulin, "Public Solidly behind Axworthy's Reforms," *Financial Post*, October 22–24, 1994, 1.
40. Therese Jennissen, "Implications for Women: The Canada Health and Social Transfer," in *The Welfare State in Canada*, ed. Blake et al., 222, 224.
41. According to Jennissen, the only CAP social assistance principle that remained in the terms of the CHST involved mobility rights, meaning "the right to an income based on need regardless of what province the person is from" (ibid., 226). See also Alan Moscovitch, "The Canada Health and Social Transfer," 107; and Keith G. Banting, "The Welfare State as Statecraft: Territorial Politics and Canadian Social Policy," in *European Social Policy: Between Fragmentation and Integration*, ed. Stephan Leibfried and Paul Pierson (Washington, D.C.: Brookings Institution, 1995), 292. It is notable that while health-care standards embodied in the Canada Health Act continued under the terms of the CHST, four out of five social assistance principles contained in CAP were discarded under the new regime.
42. Compare, for example, data in Cynthia Costello and Anne J. Stone, eds., *The American Woman, 1994–95: Where We Stand* (New York: Norton, 1994), with those in *Women in Canada: A Statistical Report* (Ottawa: Minister of Industry, 1995).
43. See, for example, Ken Battle, "The National Child Benefit," in *Canada's National Child Benefit*, ed. Durst, 38–60.
44. Little, *"No Car, No Radio, No Liquor Permit,"* 151.
45. Durst, "Phoenix or Fizzle," 15.
46. Little, *"No Car, No Radio, No Liquor Permit,"* 151.
47. See Ruth Levitas, *The Inclusive Society? Social Exclusion and New Labour* (London: Macmillan, 1998), chap. 7.
48. Tony Blair, "Introduction: My Vision for Britain," in *What Needs to Change: New Visions for Britain*, ed. Giles Radice (London: HarperCollins, 1996), 3, 6.
49. Ibid., 11.
50. Harman, as quoted in *The Guardian*, December 11, 1997, quoted in Simon Duncan and Rosalind Edwards, *Lone Mothers, Paid Work and Gendered Moral Rationalities* (London: Macmillan, 1999), 289.
51. Blair, as quoted in House of Commons Library Research Paper 19/1999 at www.parliament.uk/commons/lib/research/rp99/rp99.htm.

52. On changes to appeals procedures, see Sylvia Bashevkin, *Welfare Hot Buttons: Women, Work, and Social Policy Reform* (Toronto: University of Toronto Press, 2002).
53. Ralf Dahrendorf, "The Third Way and Liberty," *Foreign Affairs* 78:5 (September/October 1999): 16. In a 1998 review of Anthony Giddens's *The Third Way*, radical Labour MP Ken Livingstone argued that New Labour's Third Way provided "a cloak for social authoritarianism." See Ken Livingstone, "There Are More Than Three Ways," *New Statesman* (September 25, 1998): 84.

Part IV
Policy Alternatives

6.

Violating Women

Rights Abuses in the American Welfare Police State

Gwendolyn Mink

Introduction

When Americans think about welfare, they imagine Black mothers with double-digit families who make bad choices about work, men, and reproduction. These images reflect popular judgments about how recipients come to their poverty and suggest what government should do about it. Predictably, Bill Clinton's call in the early 1990s to "end welfare as we know it" was as much a call to reform recipients as it was a call to reform the welfare system. Hence, when the 1996 Personal Responsibility and Work Opportunity Reconciliation Act repealed the old welfare system, it set up a harsh new police state that subordinated recipients to a series of requirements, sanctions, and stacked incentives aimed at rectifying their personal choices and family practices.

The Temporary Assistance for Needy Families (TANF) program, the welfare system established in 1996, disciplines recipients by either stealing or impairing their basic civil rights. In exchange for welfare, TANF recipients must surrender vocational freedom, sexual privacy, and reproductive choice, as well as the right to make intimate decisions about how to be and raise a family. Ordinarily these constellations of rights enjoy strong constitutional protection and form the core of the Supreme Court's jurisprudence of (heterosexual) personhood and family,[1] but under TANF, are pressured to trade these rights for resources.[2]

The most talked-about aspect of TANF is its dramaturgy of work,[3] but TANF's foremost objective is to restore the patriarchal family. Accordingly, numerous TANF provisions promote marriage and paternal headship, while frustrating childbearing and child-raising rights outside of marriage. TANF's impositions on poor mothers' right to form and sustain their own families—as well as to avoid or exit from untenable relationships with men—proceed from stiff paternity establishment and child-support enforcement rules. According to the official U.S. House of Representatives account, TANF's "exceptionally strong paternity establishment requirements" constitute its most direct attack on nonmarital childbearing, while mandatory maternal cooperation in establishing and enforcing child-support orders impairs nonmarital child-raising.[4] If mothers do not obey these rules, they lose part or all of their families' benefits.

TANF's patriarchal solutions to welfare mothers' poverty have enjoyed bipartisan support. Democrats and Republicans fought over some of the details of the 1996 TANF legislation,[5] but both agreed that poor women with children should at least be financially tied to their children's biological fathers or, better yet, be married to them. Endangering poor single women's independent childbearing decisions by condemning their decision to raise children independently, both parties agreed that poverty policy should make father-mother family formation its cardinal principle.

The 1996 Personal Responsibility and Work Opportunity Reconciliation Act, which created TANF, spelled out policy makers' belief in the social importance of father-mother families in a preamble that recited correlations between single-mother families, and such dangers as crime, poor school performance, and intergenerational single motherhood. Declaring that "marriage is the foundation of a successful society," the act went on to establish that the purpose of welfare must be not only to provide assistance to needy families, but also to "end the dependence of needy parents on government benefits by promoting job preparation, work, and marriage'; "prevent and reduce the incidence of out-of-wedlock pregnancies"; and "encourage the formation and maintenance of two-parent families."[6] Subsequent legislation and administrative regulations strengthened TANF's founding goals through fatherhood programs, discussed furthermore that "strengthen [fathers'] ability to support a family" and that promote marriage.[7]

The TANF welfare regime backed up these interventions into poor single mothers' intimate relationships by sanctioning mothers with mandatory work outside the home if they remain single. Mothers who are married do not have to work outside the home, even though they receive welfare, because labor market work by only one parent in a two-parent family satisfies TANF's work requirement.[8] Notwithstanding a decade of rhetoric about "moving from welfare to work," the TANF regime treats wage work as the alternative to marriage, not to welfare. In short, paid employment under TANF operates as a punishment for mothers' independence.

Far from "ending dependency," the TANF regime actually fosters poor mothers' dependency on individual men. Provisions that mandate father-mother family relations assume that fathers are the best substitute for welfare. The TANF regime's refusal to invest in mothers' employment opportunities and earning power enforces this assumption, for the combination of skills hierarchies and discrimination in the labor market keeps poor mothers too poor to sustain their families on their own.[9] Moreover, the TANF regime's inattention to social supports such as transportation and child care ensures that single mothers' full-time employment will be an unaffordably expensive proposition.[10]

More than a cruel punishment for poor mothers' persistent independence, the TANF work requirement is an injury to their liberty as both mothers and workers. By pressing recipients to work outside the home for thirty hours each week, the outside work requirement forecloses TANF mothers' choice to work inside the home as caregivers for their own children. It also interferes with their independent caregiving decisions, as labor market absences due to lack of child care, for example, can lead to loss of employment—which is defined as a failure to satisfy the TANF work requirement. Furthermore, the work requirement constrains TANF mothers' choices as labor market workers, such as the choice to prepare for the labor market through education, the choice to refuse a particular job, or the choice to leave an exploitative job or hostile workplace.[11]

The TANF regime batters a host of rights, frustrating recipients' independence and ensuring their inequality. As Dionne Benson-smith argues in chapter 2 of this volume, these injuries of welfare reform are born of poverty, but lived through race. Since the 1960s, the participation of women of color in welfare has been proportionately much higher than their presence in the general population. From the 1960s to the present day, 35 to 40 percent of recipients have been African American; in 1998, 37.1 percent of TANF recipients were Black. Latina and Asian-American participation has increased over this period, as the Latino and Asian-American populations as a whole have increased. In 1998, Latina participation was 20 percent, Asian-American participation was 4.6 percent, and Native-American participation was 1.6 percent.[12]

According to contemporary reports, about two-thirds of TANF recipients are African American, Asian American, Latina, and Native American. Steeper racial disparities in welfare participation may become clear in the future, as white recipients tend to leave the rolls more rapidly than women of color or have not been enrolling at all. In New York City, for example, the number of whites on welfare declined by 57 percent between 1995 and 1998, while the number of Blacks declined by 30 percent and the number of Latinas by only 7 percent.[13] Nationwide, whites' welfare participation during this period declined by 25 percent, while African Americans' participation dropped by 17 percent and Latinas' by 9 percent. As a result, women of color increased as a percentage of TANF adults. In 24 states, women of color made up more than two-thirds of adult TANF enrollments by the end of the 1990s; in 18 of those states, they made up three-quarters or more of enrollments.[14]

In the United States, this racial distribution of welfare is the logical consequence of the racial distribution of poverty. Women of color have been and still are poorer than everyone else; single mothers of color are even more so. In 1998, when 21 percent of white single-mother families lived below the poverty line, 46 percent of African-American and 48 percent of Latina single-mother families did so.[15] The racial distribution of poverty was enforced by racism and discrimination in most walks of life. In the labor market, for example, African-American women earned 36 cents less than the white male dollar and 10 cents less than a white woman's. The wage gap for Latinas was even larger: they earned 45 percent less than white men and 19 percent less than white women.[16]

If the TANF regime's assault on poor mothers' rights wields an unmistakably disparate racial impact, it does so by imposing unmistakable constraints on poor mothers' gender practices. TANF's paternity establishment, child-support enforcement, and work requirements primarily or exclusively targeted mothers who were not married—*because* they were not married. Although the total number of nonmarital births was highest among white women, the percentage of nonmarital births was highest among women of color: 73.4 percent for non-Hispanic Black women, 91.4 percent for Latinas, and 27 percent for non-Hispanic white women.[17] Furthermore, although the total number of single-parent families was highest among whites according to data published in 2000, the percentage of single-parent families among Blacks (62.3 percent) was more than twice that among whites (26.6 percent).[18] Moreover, the percentage of Black families sustained by never-married mothers (36.5 percent) was exponentially greater than the percentage of white families (6.6 percent).[19] Finally, according to the 2000 Green Book, the poverty rate was highest among "independent families" (57.7 percent) and "cohabiting families" (58 percent) sustained by never-married mothers, among whom women of color figured disproportionately.[20]

Given the racial distribution of poverty, the presence of nonmarital mothers of color on TANF rolls remains disproportionately high. TANF's gendered provisions are therefore racialized in their effects and echo the older ideas of the Moynihan Report, as discussed earlier by Dionne Bensonsmith. Sounding the alarm against "fatherless childrearing," the TANF regime stakes itself to "the perspicacity of Moynihan's vision" that "[B]lack Americans [are] held back economically and socially in large part because their family structure [is] deteriorating."[21] And so the TANF regime exploits women of color poverty to suffocate single mothers' independence.

Women's Rights under TANF

The rights imperiled by TANF policies range from basic expectations of autonomy and privacy among civilized and respectful people, to liberty guarantees that have been deemed fundamental to constitutional citizenship. By diminishing or withholding liberty guarantees from poor single mothers who receive welfare, the TANF regime creates a welfare caste to whom constitutional principles do not apply.

One of the engines behind the 1996 welfare reform was the idea that constitutional protections won by recipients during the 1960s and early 1970s undermined recipients' responsibility and increased their "dependency." The 1996 law accordingly aimed to substitute welfare discipline for welfare rights. This involved inventing or refining program requirements to minimize participants' decisional autonomy, personal privacy, and independent personhood. Program rules not only require states to injure recipients' rights, but also require recipients to explicitly acquiesce to injury in "Personal Responsibility Contracts" they must sign in order to apply for or participate in TANF.[22]

The most visible rights abuse of the TANF regime is its impairment of recipients' vocational liberty. Mandatory work requirements obligate recipients to perform labor market work even if they are not paid for that work, as in workfare. As Leah F. Vosko demonstrates in chapter 7, TANF's "work-first" structure and philosophy further compel recipients entering the paid labor force to take the first job they are offered, even if they will not be paid a fair wage or be supplied with tolerable working conditions. Such work requirements prohibit recipients from performing family work except after hours, even though they permit recipients to perform the same work (i.e., child care) for other people's families. By compelling a particular kind and location of labor, TANF indentures recipients to the dramaturgy of work and so dictates their vocational choices.[23]

Family freedom is another right impaired by TANF program requirements, incentives, and preferences. TANF provisions tell recipients who gets to be part of their families. Paternity establishment and child-support rules require mothers to associate at least financially with biological fathers. States may excuse a mother from complying for "good cause," if this decision is seen to be "in the best interest of the child."[24] In general, however, a mother must reveal the identity of her child's father and must pursue a child-support order against him, whether or not she wants him to be financially involved in her family's life. Seventeen states require mothers to cooperate with paternity establishment and child-support enforcement while their TANF applications are pending—that is, before they receive even a dime in cash assistance.[25] Once a mother receives TANF benefits, her failure to cooperate results in an automatic 25 percent reduction in cash assistance to her family. States are permitted to go beyond this sanction and terminate welfare eligibility altogether.[26]

As TANF's implementing agency at the federal level, the U.S. Department of Health and Human Services not only enforces TANF provisions, but also enhances enforcement with additional regulations and programs. One program, the "Fatherhood Initiative," begun the Clinton administration aggressively works to improve paternity establishment rates. It claims to have contributed to the tripling of established paternities from 512,000 in fiscal year 1992 to 1.5 million in 1998.[27]

Reaching beyond mere paternity to fathers' involvement in families, Health and Human Services awarded grants and waivers to states in support of governmental, faith-based, and nonprofit initiatives such as "Parents' Fair Share" and "Partners for Fragile Families," which aim to engage fathers in the legal, emotional, and financial aspects of parenthood.[28] The department complements its strategy toward fathers with suggestions about how TANF funds can be used to promote marriage among mothers. Official federal guidelines point out that TANF block grants are "extraordinarily flexible" and allow states to *"change eligibility rules to provide incentives for single parents to marry or for two-parent families to stay together."*[29] Eligibility rules for parents who need TANF—mostly, single mothers—can include mandatory enrollment in marriage classes and couples counseling; incentives can include cash payments to TANF mothers who marry.

Legislation titled the Responsible Fatherhood Act, introduced by a Republican member of the U.S. House of Representatives from the state of Connecticut, Nancy Johnson, would amend TANF to intensify its focus on marriage. The proposed bill included a $140 million matching grant program for local projects to promote marital family formation among poor single mothers and poor noncustodial fathers. The bill also offered a $5 million award to foster a national movement of fatherhood projects and a $5 million award to a national fatherhood organization with "extensive experience in *using married couples* to deliver their program in the inner city."[30] The committee report accompanying the legislation explained that "increasing the number and percentage of American children living in two-parent families is vital if the nation is to make serious and permanent progress against poverty."[31]

In addition to requiring mothers to associate financially with fathers through child support, if not through marriage, TANF required mothers to help biological fathers develop their parental rights—their claims to access to, custody of, and decision-making over poor single mothers' children. Although child support does not in itself establish fathers' rights to children, it does afford fathers an opportunity to forge the "substantial relationship" with children that they need in court to win parental rights and custody. By compelling mothers to create parental opportunity for biological fathers, TANF's child-support cooperation rule requires mothers to participate in undermining their own parental independence.

TANF further promotes paternal opportunity through access and visitation programs that may be imposed on mothers. The Department of Health and Human Services administers TANF's provisions for access and visitation programs for fathers with a $10 million annual block grant to states to promote such programs. States may use their funds for mandatory mediation services, visitation enforcement, and developing guidelines for alternative custody arrangements.[32] Access and visitation funds may also be used for programs to encourage separating or divorcing parents to reconsider their decision, such as Iowa's mandatory education program on the impact of divorce on children.[33] The proposed Responsible Fatherhood Act would expand TANF's visitation and access provisions by authorizing funds for fatherhood projects that provide education and information to fathers about their visitation and access rights and issues.[34] These sorts of initiatives pressure mothers to open their families to biological fathers and raise the hurdles to remaining independent as mothers.

The issue at hand is not whether fathers are good for children, nor is it whether biological fathers have rights to their children. Common sense tells us that fathers can contribute positively to children's lives, both financially and emotionally. At the same time, constitutional and family law tells us that biological fathers do not enjoy rights over children merely because they share their DNA. The prerequisite to a father's right is his social, not his biological, relationship with his child—including his unrequited efforts to develop one.[35] In fact, courts grant social paternity to married fathers, even if they are not biologically related to children, on the theory that marriage establishes a social relationship to children associated with it.[36]

Although courts do enforce biological fathers' financial obligation to children even in the absence of social paternity, the obligation depends upon mothers' and children's assertion of a claim, rather than on fathers' assertion of a biological right. Moreover, the federal government historically has separated fathers' rights from their obligations, treating visitation and child support as legally separate issues. TANF visitation provisions explicitly connect these issues because "it [is] more likely for noncustodial parents to make payments of child support if they [have] either joint custody or visitation rights."[37]

The TANF regime constricts the unmarried mother's right to determine whether a social relationship with the biological father is in her child's best interest. Moreover, provisions for fatherhood actually create a social relationship between biological father and child. The TANF regime thus arms fathers with parental claims against mothers. Initiatives to restore fathers' "economic provider role" further strengthen their claims regarding children, as fathers' superior earning power makes paternal custody a real threat. Accordingly, the TANF regime's ultimate threat to independent motherhood rests in each mother's potential loss of her children.

In addition to compromising rights of intimate association, TANF requirements for paternity establishment and child-support enforcement also suspend sexual privacy. Although only consensual heterosexual sex between adults is shielded by privacy under reigning jurisprudence, even that partial right is withheld from unmarried mothers who seek welfare. As Leah F. Vosko's discussion in the next chapter shows, mandatory paternity establishment and child-support provisions require a mother to identify her child's biological father to be eligible for welfare. These provisions single out nonmarital mothers for scrutiny and punishment, as paternity is automatically established at birth if a mother is married. A mother who is not married, or who does not want anything to do with her child's biological father, must nevertheless provide welfare officials with information about him. TANF thus forces an unmarried mother to maintain enough of an association with her child's biological father to inform on his whereabouts, even against her wishes or best judgment. If a mother does not know the identity of her child's biological father or does not want to reveal it, she must submit to interrogation by the government about her sex life, so that the government can identify paternal suspects.

Even under TANF's predecessor, the Aid to Families with Dependent Children program, paternity establishment rules compromised recipients' privacy. To obtain the information they sought, welfare officials and courts required independent mothers to answer such questions as, "How many sexual partners have you had? ... With whom did you have sex before you got pregnant? ... How often did you have sex? ... Where did you have sex? ... When did you have sex?"[38] TANF encouraged more aggressive and systematic intrusion into recipients' sex lives. First, states were required to punish noncooperating mothers with benefits cuts. Second, mothers were forced to sign child support income over to the state as a condition of receiving welfare. And third, the Clinton administration offered incentives and services to boost paternity establishment rates.

Besides sexual privacy, TANF injures other reproductive rights when it interferes in women's childbearing decisions. For example, the TANF regime let stand state-level policies that withheld benefits from additional children born to mothers who were already enrolled on welfare. Beginning in the early 1990s, many states promulgated these "family cap" policies after securing waivers from federal welfare standards under the Bush and Clinton administrations. The family cap impairs reproductive rights because it punishes and deters a recipient's choice to complete a pregnancy.

TANF further injures reproductive rights through the use of "illegitimacy bonuses."[39] This bonus is paid to the five states that most successfully reduce the number of nonmarital births without raising their abortion rates. It offers states an incentive to discourage conception by unmarried women—by offering cash awards to women who use Norplant birth control devices, for example. Sending a further message against having children outside marriage, the TANF regime funds states that offer abstinence-only education programs. These are required to teach women not to have sex, let alone babies, until they are "economically self-sufficient." States may devolve abstinence-only programs to private grantees, including church-based groups that treat abstinence as a matter of "values" and "sexual morality."[40]

As a corollary to abstinence education, TANF calls for invigorated statutory rape prosecutions—underscoring the abstinence message with a threat of criminal sanctions where teenagers are involved.[41] As a poor minor woman's nonmarital pregnancy is proof of sex before economic self-sufficiency, the threatened prosecution of nonmarital sex involving welfare recipients is another intrusion on poor single mothers' independence, including on their reproductive autonomy. When threats fail to deter sex and pregnancy, TANF's prohibition on assistance to unmarried teenage mothers who are not living with a responsible adult delivers unambiguous punishment.

In short, the TANF regime controls its subjects through a range of proscriptions and punishments. Each proscription and punishment injures poor single mothers' rights to mother independently—of either men or the government. Ultimately, the TANF regime assails poor single women's right to be mothers at all. The final blow to this right is delivered by child welfare and adoption provisions that speed and ease the process of terminating poor mothers' custody of children.

Although the TANF legislation repealed the income entitlement that had belonged to poor mothers and their children, it continued children's entitlement to be removed from unfit parents and placed in foster care. I have no quarrel with children's entitlement to protective services. However, the discretion delegated to child welfare workers permits them to deploy children's entitlement to foster care as a weapon of welfare discipline against their mothers. A mother who did not comply with work requirements, for example, might be deemed an unfit provider. A mother who left her child alone to go to a job interview because she could not find child care could be deemed an unfit caregiver. If she were sanctioned off welfare, had to take a low-wage job, or exhausted her eligibility, a mother might not be able to pay the rent or feed her children. These kinds of circumstances could lead to a finding that she was neglectful. A "neglectful" mother may lose custody of her child, or she may come under intensive supervision by government.

Indeed, official TANF guidelines specifically encourage states to scrutinize recipients for possible unfit parenting. The TANF regime mandates sanctions against recipients who do not meet work requirements, do not cooperate in establishing paternity, or do not cooperate in enforcing child-support orders. Sanction penalties vary among states. They range from reducing an individual mother's benefit the first time she fails to meet her work requirement, to a federally mandated reduction in benefits when a mother fails to cooperate with paternity establishment and child-support enforcement, to terminating a family's TANF assistance altogether.[42] As a practical matter, sanctioned families frequently also lose their Medicaid health benefits, even though they remain entitled to receive these. Accordingly, TANF penalties not only breed material vulnerability, but also medically endanger families.[43]

Health and Human Services guidelines stipulate that welfare monies may be used to "screen families who have been sanctioned under TANF" to determine whether children are at risk of child abuse or neglect. Mothers who do not want child support, who do not want to identify biological fathers, or who cannot meet the thirty hours per week work requirement thus come under suspicion as abusive or neglectful parents. Mothers who exercise their rights and independent judgment are held to account for the consequences of TANF's brutal rules. If a mother's children are found to be at risk due to sanctions, TANF funds may be used to provide "case management services" to "cure" the mother's noncompliance with TANF rules.[44]

TANF mothers who lose their benefits—like employed single

mothers whose wages are too low to pay for housing, food, or medical care—may surrender their children to foster care. Occasionally, a mother might do so voluntarily, until she can get back on her feet. Alternatively, child welfare workers might pressure a mother to do so. The 1997 Adoption and Safe Families Act threatens mothers who have lost their children to foster care with the permanent termination of their parental rights. Designed to accelerate and increase foster care adoptions, the act requires child welfare workers to consider terminating parental rights if a child has been in foster care for fifteen out of the previous twenty-two months.[45] In the years following enactment of the adoption law, adoptions increased significantly, from 28,000 in 1996 to 46,000 in 1999.[46] We do not yet have hard evidence directly linking the rise in adoptions with recipients' loss of children. However, with a time limit on parental rights shorter than even the federal time limit on welfare, the adoption law hovers within the TANF regime as the ultimate solution to independent motherhood.

Ensuring Independence

TANF rules and regulations enforce inequality by depriving recipients of rights that other citizens continue to enjoy. In turn, TANF ensures inequality by withdrawing the right to receive benefits—by ending the entitlement to welfare. In its most draconian innovation by far, TANF ended the old welfare system's income security guarantee for poor mothers and their children and replaced it with time-limited, discretionary cash assistance.[47] Consistent with Sylvia Bashevkin's argument in chapter 5 about the erosion of Anglo-American social citizenship, women's rights abuses within the TANF regime strip recipients of their autonomy as women and as mothers. The end of the welfare entitlement exacerbates the injuries of the TANF welfare regime, since eligible mothers who are turned away from TANF and mothers who exhaust their eligibility due to time limits are forced into deepening dependency—on charity, men, and jobs they dare not refuse.

One measure of the endangered economic status of mothers who need welfare is the persistence of poverty even among mothers who have left welfare for the labor market. Three years after leaving welfare, the median income among employed former welfare recipients in the United States was only $10,924 in 1999—well below the poverty line of $14,150 for a family of three. In many former TANF families, income is so low or so tenuous that families must skip meals, go hungry, use charity food banks, or apply for emergency food assistance. In New Jersey in 1999, 47.9 percent of former recipients who were employed reported that they could not provide adequate food for their children. In Illinois, 63 percent of recipients who participated in the paid labor force reported similar problems.[48]

The main reason for the persistence of poverty among former TANF recipients was that they moved primarily into low-wage and contingent jobs without benefits, losing access to federal Food Stamps vouchers and Medicaid health insurance, and surrendered as much as 25 percent of their paychecks to child care. The persistence of poverty led many policy makers to pursue a "next step" in welfare reform. An emergent consensus suggested that poor single mothers need a wage supplement, after all—in the form of a father's income. A related consensus maintained that if welfare reform fell short, it was because too few recipients got married.[49]

This ominous "next step" in welfare reform was revealed at the legislative level in "fatherhood initiatives" that proposed to enhance paternal wages and the paternal role. Fatherhood proposals were espoused in various ideological quarters: by major party presidential candidates in 2000; by Republican Nancy Johnson and Democrat Benjamin Cardin, respectively chair and ranking member of the House of Representatives Ways and Means Subcommittee on Human Resources; and by Democratic member of Congress Jesse Jackson Jr.

The Johnson-Cardin fatherhood bill passed the House of Representatives in the fall of 2000, as part of the Child Support Distribution Act. The bill offered fathers incentives to enter poor mothers' families. For example, it promoted forgiving child support payments owed by men who became residential fathers and enhanced fathers' earning power through job training and "career-advancing education." The bill aimed to improve fathers' ability to meet their financial responsibilities; it also tracked nonmarital fathers into various social service programs that encourage marriage.⁵⁰ These incentives to fathers imposed substantial pressures on mothers, for it is mothers, not fathers, who must obey TANF rules and suffer the consequences of time limits. Fathers get the "carrots," to borrow the jargon of conservative welfare reform advocate Charles Murray, while mothers get the "sticks."

Jesse Jackson Jr.'s bill duplicated the Johnson-Cardin bill in many respects, including in its name. Jackson's proposed Responsible Fatherhood Act would amend TANF to add more explicit language about the virtues of marriage and the importance of fathers. Many of the Johnson-Cardin provisions to support a national fatherhood campaign and to provide block grants to states for fatherhood programs also appeared in the Jackson bill. Perhaps most astounding, much of the rhetoric that shaped earlier Republican welfare reform initiatives (including the 1996 Personal Responsibility and Work Opportunity Reconciliation Act) was repeated in the preamble to the Jackson bill. To wit, section 2 of the bill, which reports Congress's "findings," asserts:

> children who live without contact with their biological father are ... (A) five times more likely to live in poverty; (B) more likely to bring weapons and drugs into the classroom; (C) twice as likely to commit crime; (D) twice as likely to drop out of school; (E) twice as likely to be abused; (F) more likely to commit suicide; (G) more than twice as likely to abuse alcohol or drugs; and (H) more likely to become pregnant as teenagers.

Echoing the 1965 Moynihan Report, discussed by Dionne Bensonsmith in chapter 2 of this book, the preamble continues, "Violent criminals are overwhelmingly males who grew up without fathers and the best predictor of crime in a community is the percentage of absent father households." The preamble concludes, "States should be encouraged, not restricted, from implementing programs that provide support for responsible fatherhood, promote marriage, and increase the incidence of marriage."⁵¹

Thirty years into the second wave of U.S. feminism, even progressives like Jesse Jackson Jr. were shamelessly promoting heterosexual, two-parent, father-headed family life as the solution to mothers' poverty. Worse, they were making their case at the expense of poor mothers, who were blamed for countless social ills associated with poverty. The costs of this analysis included the odious moralistic interventions permitted or required by welfare law to encourage marriage or marriagelike financial coupling between biological parents. They also included the punishment of full-time work outside the home for mothers who remained persistently single.

Welfare payments in the United States originated early in the last century to recognize that lone mothers bore sole responsibility for both supporting their families and caring for them. The idea behind what were then called mothers' pensions was to relieve single mothers' income-earning burden by subsidizing their caring work, so that they would have the time and the cash to attend to their children. Over the course of the twentieth century, the expectation that welfare should at least partially support the caring work of single mothers dissipated, amid jeers against single women of color having children at all.

The original U.S. welfare program posed many problems for women's equality: It assumed mother's domesticity, intervened in cultural and other family decisions, and applied racist and moralistic criteria to assess the worthiness of potential recipients. At the same time, early-twentieth-century welfare noticed the nexus between women's poverty and women's caring work in families. This was the first step toward building a concept of gender equality based not only on some women's escape from the historic work of their gender, but also on other women's winning full social and economic recognition for that work.

Despite this potential, the interconnectedness among poverty, caregiving, and inequality never received wide or focused attention in the United States. Although policies emerged to provide income assistance to family caregivers, those policies were either stingy and marginal, or their eligibility rules were extremely narrow so that beneficiaries were relatively few. In addition, to the extent that welfare and other policies assisted family caregivers, they did so primarily to protect children's interests, rather than to compensate mothers' work or to promote mothers' equality.

Unlike the West European situation described in chapters 1 and 3 by Selma Sevenhuijsen and Jane Jenson, most feminists in the United States have been leery of taking up the cause of women's caregiving work—preferring to promote women's equality as labor market workers, rather than to risk a return to compulsory domesticity. In response to the TANF regime, however, some feminists have begun not only to resist welfare's moral discipline, but also to reconceive welfare as caregivers' income.[52] The idea is that what caregivers—usually, mothers—do for their families is work. Moreover, it is work that is indispensable not only to a mother's own family, but also to her community, the economy, and the polity.

Far from a sign of dependence on government, a caregivers' income would provide mothers with economic means *in their own right*. It would promote equality in father-mother relations, both because it would unmask the economic value of mothers' side of the sexual division of labor and because it would enable mothers to exit unhappy, subordinating, or violent relations with the fathers of their children. A caregiving allowance would also nurture equality among citizens by establishing that it is not only market work that should earn a living wage, but also the caring work upon which the market depends for workers that demands remuneration. In turn, a caregivers' income would promote equality among women—between middle-class, married caregivers who enjoy social and political support when they choose to work inside the home raising children and poor unmarried caregivers, for whom welfare policy now compels a choice of wages over caring.

Improved economic rewards and social supports for women's work outside the home are necessary companions to a social wage for their work inside the home. Women must not be pressured into giving care at home by the low returns they receive for labor market participation. Just as important, they must not be pressed to forsake care work by the threat of destitution. In combination with labor market reforms, a caregivers' income would indemnify women's—and even men's—vocational choices. "Making work pay," both in the home and in the labor market, would help to combat the persistent poverty of single-mother families, without pinning family security to fathers' responsibility.

Rethinking welfare as an income owed to caregivers would help to lessen the severe material vulnerabilities facing single mothers. As well, it would exhume the rights suffocated by both poverty and the current welfare system. Once welfare mothers are understood to be poor at least in part because their family caregiving work is unremunerated, then the focus of welfare prescriptions can shift from how to reform disadvantaged caregivers to how to cure their poverty.

The idea that a caregiver's income is due because the family caregiver *works* would rescue single mothers from racialized stigmas of sloth, immorality, and dependency that have nourished punitive and behavioral welfare reforms. The idea that a caregiver's income is due because the caregiver is an independent worker would defend single mothers from patriarchal pressures to rely on individual men. The idea that a caregiver's income is due so that single mothers can make independent choices about partners, children, and work would revive women's rights as the rights of all women.

Notes

Earlier versions of the material appeared in the *Annals* of the American Academy of Political and Social Science 577 (September 2001): 79–93.

1. For details of the PRWORA legislation, see Gwendolyn Mink, *Welfare's End* (Ithaca, N.Y.: Cornell University Press, 1998), chap. 1.
2. *Legal Services Corporation v. Velazquez*, No. 99-603 (2000). U.S. Supreme Court.
3. Frances Fox Piven and Richard Cloward, *Regulating the Poor: The Functions of Public Welfare* (New York: Pantheon, 1971), chap. 11, 346, 381, 395.
4. U.S. House of Representatives, Ways and Means Committee, 106th Cong., *2000 Green Book: Overview of Entitlement Programs*, 2000, 1530.
5. House Democrats proposed alternatives to the Republicans' bill in both 1995 and 1996, for example. In 1995, the Democrats offered a substitute bill that imposed work requirements and time limits, but preserved the welfare entitlement. In 1996, they proposed a bipartisan substitute that ended the entitlement and sanctioned mothers who did not cooperate with paternity and child-support rules. It also provided for mandatory and voluntary programs to enhance fathers' access to children.
6. Public Law 104-193, Title I.

7. The 1999 Welfare-to-Work Amendments loosened rules that governed the eligibility of noncustodial parents for services. Noncustodial fathers became eligible if they were unemployed, or underemployed or had difficulty paying child-support obligations; if their children had received TANF benefits during the preceding year; if they were eligible to receive Food Stamps, Supplemental Security Income, Medicaid, or Children's Health Insurance; and if they entered into a personal responsibility contract regarding paternity establishment, child support, and improving their earning power. Eligibility for Welfare-to-Work services is not an entitlement—that is, it is not guaranteed to all who meet the program's criteria. Hence, fathers' increased access to services takes services away from mothers on the brink of reaching welfare time limits. See U.S. Department of Labor, "The 1999 Welfare-to-Work Amendments," http://wtw.doleta.gov/laws-regs/99amendsum.htm. As of late 2000, the U.S. Senate was considering a House-passed "Responsible Fatherhood" bill that aimed to "increase marriage, improve parenting, and increase the income of fathers." See U.S. House of Representatives, Committee on Ways and Means, Child Support Distribution Act of 2000: Report to Accompany H.R. 4678, Rept. 106–793, pt. I, 106th Cong., 2nd Sess., 26 July 2000, 17.
8. P.L. 104-193, sec. 407(c)(1)(B); *2000 Green Book*, 357. A two-parent family is required to work thirty-five hours weekly (as compared to a thirty hour/week requirement for single parents), unless the family receives federally funded child care. A two-parent family that sends its child or children to federally funded child care must perform fifty-five hours of labor market work weekly—which permits married mothers to work part time.
9. See, for example, Gregory Acs, Norma Coe, Keith Watson, and Robert I. Lerman, *Does Work Pay? An Analysis of the Work Incentives under TANF* (Washington, D.C.: Urban Institute, 1998); Robert Moffitt and Jennifer Roff, "The Diversity of Welfare Leavers," in *Welfare, Children, and Families: A Three-City Study*, Johns Hopkins University, Working Paper 00-01 (October 12, 2000); and Wider Opportunities for Women, "Job Retention and Advancement Issues" (October 25, 2000).
10. For example, the legislation that created TANF also ended the child-care entitlement for welfare recipients. On the discouraging and impoverishing costs of employment for many recipients, see Kathryn Edin and Laura Lein, *Making Ends Meet: How Single Mothers Survive Welfare and Low-Wage Work* (New York: Russell Sage Foundation, 1997).
11. For key work provisions, see P.L. 104-193, Title I, sec. 407(a)(1); 407(c)(2)(B); 407(e)(1).
12. U.S. Department of Health and Human Services, Administration for Children and Families, "Characteristics and Financial Circumstances of TANF Recipients," table 12; *2000 Green Book*, 438.

13. Jason deParle, "Shrinking Welfare Rolls Leave Record High Share of Minorities," *New York Times*, July 24, 1998, A1.
14. *2000 Green Book*, table 7–29, 439.
15. United States Census Bureau, "Poverty Thresholds in 1998 by Size of Family and Number of Related Children under 18 Years" (Washington, D.C., 1999), cited in Women of Color Resource Center, *Working Hard, Staying Poor: Women and Children in the Wake of Welfare "Reform"* (Berkeley: Women of Color Resource Center, 2000), 25.
16. Katharine G. Abraham, commissioner of labor statistics, Testimony before the U.S. Senate, Committee on Health, Education, Labor and Pensions, 106th Cong. , 2nd sess., 8 June 2000.
17. *2000 Green Book*, 1238, 1521.
18. *2000 Green Book*, table G-4, 1239.
19. Ibid.
20. *2000 Green Book*, table G-11, 1246.
21. *2000 Green Book*, 1519.
22. State Policy Documentation Project, "Findings in Brief: TANF Applications," March 3, 2000, and "Personal Responsibility Contracts: Obligations," June 1999, http://www.spdp.org/tanf/applications/appsumm.htm.
23. Mink, *Welfare's End*, chap. 4.
24. *2000 Green Book*, 470.
25. State Policy Documentation Project, "Pending Application Requirements," May 1999, http://www.spdp.org/tanf/applications/.
26. P.L. 104-193, Title I, sec. 408(a)(2).
27. U.S. Department of Health and Human Services, "HHS Fatherhood Initiative Fact Sheet," June 17, 2000.
28. U.S. Department of Health and Human Services, "HHS's Fatherhood Initiative: Improving Opportunities for Low-Income Fathers," 2000.
29. U.S. Department of Human Services, Administration for Children and Families, Office of Family Assistance, Program Announcement Form, "Helping Families Achieve Self-Sufficiency: A Guide for Funding Services for Children and Families through the TANF Program," http://www.acf. dhhs.gov/programs/ofa/funds2.htm (pp. 3 and 19 of 24), italics added.
30. H.R. 4678, Title V, Subtitle B, sec. 511(c)(2)(c), U.S. House of Representatives, 106th Cong., 2nd sess., italics added.
31. Child Support Distribution Act of 2000: Report to Accompany H.R. 4678, U.S. House of Representatives, Committee on Ways and Means.
32. U.S. Department of Health and Human Services, "HHS Fatherhood Initiative Fact Sheet."
33. Stanley Bernard, "Responsible Fatherhood and Welfare: How States Can Use the New Law to Help Children," *Children and Welfare Reform*, Issue Brief 4 (New York: National Center for Children in Poverty, Columbia University, 1998), 9–10.

34. Child Support Distribution Act of 2000: Report, 42.
35. See, for example, *Lehr v. Robertson* 463 U.S. 248 (1983) 248, 256, 261–62.
36. *Michael H. v. Gerald D.* 491 U.S. 110 (1988).
37. *2000 Green Book*, 469.
38. Lisa Kelly, "If Anybody Asks You Who I Am: An Outsider's Story of the Duty to Establish Paternity," *Yale Journal of Law and Feminism* 6 (1994): 303–304.
39. P.L. 104-193, sec. 403(a)(2). The 1997 Balanced Budget Act defined the illegitimacy ratio as the relationship of nonmarital births to all births.
40. See, for example, Pierre Toussaint/Human Services Division, abstinence education grant proposal to the State of Florida; Empowering the Vision, abstinence education grant proposal to the State of Florida. Thanks to Debra Rosen for investigating how abstinence education funds are being used.
41. P.L. 104-193, sec. 402(a)(1)(v).
42. For a summary of work-related sanctions, see State Policy Documentation Project, "Sanctions for Noncompliance with Work Activities," http://www.spdp.org/tanf/sanctions/sanctions_findings.htm.
43. M. Robin Dion and LaDonna Pavetti, "Access to and Participation in Medicaid and the Food Stamp Program: A Review of the Recent Literature" (Washington, D.C.: Mathematica Policy Research, March 7, 2000), 15–17.
44. "Helping Families Achieve Self-Sufficiency," 19.
45. Adoption Promotion Act of 1997, U.S. House of Representatives, 105th Cong., 1st sess, H.R. 867.
46. U.S. Department of Health and Human Services, HHS News, "HHS Awards Adoption Bonuses and Grants" (Washington, D.C., September 20, 2000).
47. The TANF law does not prohibit *states* from providing a state-level entitlement. Five states (Alaska, Hawaii, Maryland, Rhode Island, and Vermont) have provided such an entitlement to cash assistance for poor families that meet the various conditions for welfare participation, such as child-support cooperation and mandatory work outside the home. State Policy Documentation Project, "Findings in Brief: Entitlement to Benefits," http://www.spdp.org/tanf/entitlement/cash_assistance_entitlement_summlist.htm.
48. Chicago Urban League and UIC Center for Urban Economic Development, *Living with Welfare Reform: A Survey of Low Income Families in Illinois* (Chicago, January 2000); Study Group on Work, Poverty and Welfare, *Assessing Work First: What Happens after Welfare?* (New Jersey, June 1999), as quoted in Women of Color Resource Center, *Working Hard, Staying Poor*, 19. On the argument that caseload declines have far exceeded declines in poverty, see Sandra Danziger, Mary Corcoran, Sheldon Danziger, and Colleen Heflin, "Work, Income, and Material Hardship after Welfare Reform," *Journal of Consumer Affairs* 34 (2000): 6ff.
49. Of the TANF cases closed between October 1997 and September

1998, only 0.4 percent were due to marriage. See "Characteristics and Financial Circumstances of TANF Recipients, Fiscal Year 1998," table 31. Although the annual percentage increase in the number of single-parent (primarily mother-only) families decreased, the number continued to rise. Likewise, the number and percentage of never-married-mother families increased.
50. H.R. 4678, Title V, Subtitle A, sec. 501(a) and 501(b).
51. "The Responsible Fatherhood Act of 2000," Jesse Jackson Jr. sponsor. U.S. House of Representatives, 106th Cong., 2nd sess., H.R. 4671. Introduced on June 15, 2000.
52. Women's Committee of 100/Project 2002, *An Immodest Proposal: Rewarding Women's Work to End Poverty* (March 23, 2000).

7.
Mandatory "Marriage" or Obligatory Waged Work

Social Assistance and Single Mothers in Wisconsin and Ontario

Leah F. Vosko

Introduction

Among feminist scholars, the single mother is frequently cast as the barometer of the welfare state.[1] The kinds of supports to which she is entitled not only reflect the strength or weakness of her social citizenship rights, but also are indicative of the nature and organization of social protection in a given regime. As a category of recipient, the single mother is subject to extensive scrutiny in social assistance policies, which frequently convey highly gendered notions of "dependence" and "independence" (see Selma Sevenhuijsen's discussion in chapter 1 of this volume). In the current period, therefore, the changing shape of social assistance policy is a sound predictor of the direction, content, and gendered character of welfare state change.

Feminist inquiries into social assistance, especially those that dissect foundational concepts and understandings surrounding the welfare state and relate them to prevalent policies and practices, shed valuable light on the shifting meaning of social citizenship. Many scholars working in this stream reject the gendered assumptions that inform emergent social assistance policies in the United States and Canada. They argue that the single mother should have the right to live independently and, therefore, be free to opt out of the nuclear family and still retain access to a full range of social benefits and entitlements that enable her to escape poverty and provide for her children.[2] Such sentiments lead a growing number of feminist writers to advance alternative proposals, ranging from paid leaves from employment and care allowances to collectivized child care, all aimed at securing basic social citizenship rights for the single mother.

Recent developments in social assistance policy in Wisconsin and Ontario conflict fundamentally with feminist objectives and alternatives.[3] A complex and contradictory process of restructuring is underway in both of these subnational jurisdictions, arguably the two most developed workfare regimes in the United States and Canada, respectively. This process threatens to leave single mothers seeking social assistance with essentially two options. Their first option is to secure financial assistance by attaching themselves to a man, either via measures like paternity establishment and child-support retrieval mandated by the state or through nuclear family formation. As Gwendolyn Mink argues in chapter 6, this option reflects a conservative "family values" agenda.[4] Their second option, which only materializes after privatized forms of support are exhausted, involves mandatory work in exchange for welfare under a multitiered scheme of workfare-style programs. This alternative is rooted in a narrow conception of "self-sufficiency" or "independence," linked to labor force participation and tied to the increasingly common objective of decreasing women's reliance on state support, especially in welfare regimes influenced by a neoliberal economic paradigm.

This chapter explores the conditions under which single mothers can access a range of social citizenship rights available in Wisconsin and Ontario. It proceeds in three parts, the first of which sketches developments at the federal level in the United States and Canada that influence new directions in social assistance policy at the state or provincial level. The next part examines changes in legislation, regulations, and policies in Wisconsin and Ontario that introduce mandatory work requirements for categories of social assistance recipients, including single mothers of young children. These two strands of investigation identify the combination of conservative policies, consistent with a "family values" agenda that encourages particular social norms and family forms, and neoliberal policies that exact "self-sufficiency" through waged work in each jurisdiction, focusing on their implications for the single mother. Building on this analysis, the third part explores one potential alternative policy scenario—the introduction of a care allowance or caregiver stream directed at single mothers—and touches on two other alternatives, collectivized child care and parental leave. Paradoxically, some feminist scholars (including Gwendolyn Mink in chapter 6 of this volume) support care allowances in principle, even though these allowances have the capacity to reinforce the negative consequences for single mothers that flow from workfare regimes in Wisconsin and Ontario.[5]

Developments in Federal Social Assistance Policy

The United States and Canada followed distinct paths in federal social assistance policy until the late twentieth century.[6] Early in the century, the United States adopted a means-tested model of poor relief, which was first available exclusively to children, but was subsequently extended to families with dependent children. For decades, the Aid to Families with Dependent Children program (AFDC) stood as the primary vehicle for families with children to access social assistance.[7] In contrast, Canada followed a needs-tested model rooted in the assumption that the needs of citizens varied, based on individual circumstances. Like the United States, Canada initiated its social assistance approach based partly on subnational experiments with mothers' allowances. Canadian social assistance eventually included single people, making its coverage more extensive.

Cross-national differences persisted well into the 1960s. The Canada Assistance Plan (CAP), introduced in 1966, set up a system of federal- provincial cost-sharing that provided for comprehensive and relatively generous social provision. CAP brought together Old Age Security, Blind Persons' Assistance, Disabled Persons' Assistance, and Unemployment Assistance under the same umbrella. It also introduced three core principles that made social assistance programs accessible to a wide group of citizens: cash assistance would be available to anyone in need, no residency requirements could be imposed, and persons denied support had the right to appeal. As well, under the terms of CAP, provinces could not make work requirements a condition for receiving social assistance.

Sharp differences between U.S. and Canadian social assistance policy did not persist for very long, however. In Canada, pressures on the federal government to cut back on social programs grew as early as the late 1970s, but took hold during the next two decades. The precise causes of a definitive shift toward work incentives in these decades are difficult to ascertain, particularly in contrast to those operating in the United States, where a more predictable and incremental process unfolded.[8] Still, federal social assistance policies in North America began to converge in the 1980s and 1990s and generated similar gendered outcomes.

Several developments at the federal level in both countries helped to fuel changes in Wisconsin and Ontario. In the United States, President Clinton announced a campaign to "end welfare as we know it" in 1992. His plan aimed to give welfare recipients a two-year time limit to reestablish their financial "self-sufficiency." Clinton's proposals were eventually overtaken by Republican demands coming out of that party's 1994 "Contract with America" platform, which included provisions even more stringent than those proposed by Clinton.[9] In 1996, Clinton signed the Personal Responsibility and Work Opportunity Reconciliation Act (PRWORA), which created a new program, known as Temporary Assistance for Needy Families (TANF), to replace AFDC.

PRWORA allowed the federal government to transfer AFDC cost-sharing to a block grant that would reduce federal spending by $55 billion over six years. Through TANF, it introduced four important changes to the provision of social assistance:

- a five-year lifetime limit on welfare, allowing states to exempt up to 20 percent of their caseload for hardship reasons and to set shorter time limits if desired;
- the requirement that welfare recipients begin working within two years of receiving welfare and that half of all single-parent families work thirty hours a week by 2002;
- reductions in spending on food stamps by $28 billion over six years, achieved partly by restricting them for able-bodied individuals without children to three months in any three-year period unless they were working part time;
- the elimination of federal aid (including Medicaid) and cash welfare for immigrants for five years after attaining citizenship.[10]

The ultimate aim of PRWORA was to reduce federal spending by setting time limits on benefits, shifting program delivery to individual states, and ending a legally enforceable right of individuals to collect social assistance.

In addition to these changes, PRWORA introduced measures designed to regulate the conduct of single mothers on social assistance. As detailed by Gwendolyn Mink in chapter 6, lone mothers had to disclose the paternity of their children (Section 608[a]1), teenage parents had to live with an adult (Section 608[a]4 and 5), and states were offered incentives to reduce out-of-wedlock births without increasing abortion rates. These measures reflected the general tone of the legislation, which began with a preamble stating that marriage is the foundation of a successful society, marriage is an essential institution that promotes the interests of children, and the promotion of responsible fatherhood and motherhood is integral to the well-being of children.[11]

As a unit, PRWORA aimed to

- provide assistance to families so that children may be cared for in their own homes or in the homes of relatives;
- end dependence of needy parents on government benefits by promoting job preparation, work, and marriage;
- prevent and reduce the incidence of out-of-wedlock pregnancies and compel states to establish annual numerical goals for preventing and reducing the incidence of these pregnancies;
- encourage the formation and maintenance of two-parent families.[12]

Since little effort was made to use gender-neutral language in the federal legislation, the text of PRWORA was filled with rhetoric about "individualized dependency."[13] As Dionne Bensonsmith and Gwendolyn Mink suggest in chapters 2 and 6, the 1996 welfare reform bill was also underpinned by highly racialized images of the single mother.

The replacement of CAP by the Canada Health and Social Transfer (CHST) in 1996 appeared to be, at first glance, less punitive and more gender-neutral. The CHST rolled federal funding for social assistance together with federal income transfers to finance health and education programs into one block grant.

No federal welfare standards were retained in the legislation, except that the CHST contained a prohibition on provincial residency requirements for the receipt of social assistance.

Although the CHST was widely interpreted as a signal of social policy retrenchment, its provisions were frequently portrayed as less severe than those introduced in the same year in the United States. For example, Gerard Boychuk argues that "while block-funding in Canada does not stipulate any minimum national standards in social assistance provision (with the exception of the ban on residency requirements), neither does it stipulate maximum national standards of provision as block-funding now does in United States."[14] Hence, according to Boychuk, social assistance reform was more extreme in the United States, where the federal government set maximum payments and lifetime limits. An absence of maximums in Canada, however, in no way *prevents* downward harmonization in social assistance policy.

Provisions of the 1999 Social Union Framework Agreement, or SUFA, between the Canadian federal government and ten provinces underscored the potential for downward harmonization in social assistance, or at least considerable territorial variation because of increased provincial autonomy. On the one hand, SUFA was significant because it reasserted the principle that governments would provide assistance for people in need, a feature that was integral to CAP, but was rescinded in the CHST. On the other hand, SUFA lacked national standards and paved the way for broad provincial variation in the delivery of both social assistance spending programs and newer tax-based child benefits. Under the terms of the post-SUFA Canada Child Tax Benefit, for example, provinces were permitted to claw back social assistance by the same amount as the tax benefit, to provide incentives for low-income families to work for pay. Mechanisms to check provincial accountability were absent, giving provinces like Ontario the sole responsibility to shape the directions of social assistance.

Unlike PRWORA and TANF, which are visibly gendered and racialized policies, the CHST and SUFA seem gender-neutral on their face. Yet the absence of explicitly gendered provisions does not amount to gender-neutral consequences. No formal rewards for marriage exist under the CHST. Nor are there are financial rewards for provinces that reduce "illegitimate" births. Work requirements are implicitly permitted, but *not* mandated under the terms of the CHST. Thus, Canadian definitions of "self-sufficiency" and "independence" were by no means fixed. Nevertheless, single mothers formed a very significant group of female social assistance recipients in Canada in the 1990s. As Katherine Scott observes, "in dollar terms, cuts to social assistance ... have the biggest impact on lone parents" and, as a result, lone-parent families headed by women have a high risk of poverty.[15]

Scott's figures suggest that single mothers in Canada rank among the most disadvantaged of those who are on social assistance, partly because of the introduction of the CHST. Furthermore, Canadian provinces, like U.S. states, enjoyed greater discretion over the design and content of social assistance policies in 1996 and following, with significant direction from, but limited accountability to, their respective federal governments (see Sylvia Bashevkin's discussion in chapter 5). The flexibility built into new U.S. and Canadian federal laws, regulations, and policies also had the capacity to give greater influence to conservative "family values" and neoliberal economic interests, thus facilitating harsher treatment of single mothers in both countries.

Restructuring Social Assistance in Wisconsin and Ontario

The powerful gendered logic apparent in social assistance initiatives in Wisconsin and Ontario was propelled by the complex and contradictory, but, in many respects, overlapping, objectives of conservative "family values" proponents and the larger neoliberal paradigm increasingly pervasive in the United States and Canada. In both Wisconsin and Ontario, subnational governments constructed an either/or scenario for the single mother that affected the circumstances under which she may procreate and raise her children. Both W-2, Wisconsin's welfare-to-work program, and Ontario Works, Ontario's equivalent, had strong gendered underpinnings. Each program penalized pregnant women on assistance. Each forced single mothers unattached to a male breadwinner to engage in waged work or a narrow set of equivalents. At the same time, both constructed attachment to a man as a reason for denying the single mother an independent entitlement to assistance.

The desire of both governments to remove state support from single mothers was evident in the objectives of social assistance legislation, which, in one instance, cast "marriage as the foundation of a successful society" (Wisconsin) and, in the other, favored any measure designed to increase familial or community responsibility (Ontario). It was, however, in policy and program design that the idea that the problems of the single mother stemmed primarily from the fact she was not "properly" dependent upon a man assumed its sharpest expression. This idealized notion of female dependency permeated policies on eligibility, benefit rates, and directives governing the conduct of pregnant single women.

Measures reflecting conservative ideas about the proper role of "the family" had a significant presence in Wisconsin, where work requirements for single mothers with infants over twelve weeks old made social assistance virtually unattainable to her, especially where quality child care was not readily available. A particular family form was not simply encouraged; it was effectively required, since the costs of single parenthood were so high.[16] Penalties for women having children while on assistance, through the withholding of additional payments for extra children, along with paternity-acknowledgment measures, reflected the strong influence of conservative "family values" in Wisconsin. In turn, these provisions undermined single mothers' ability to be sole custodians of their children and to maintain autonomous households, regardless of the nature of their labor force attachment.

In their respective federal contexts, Wisconsin and Ontario represented prototypes of a particular sort: each subnational jurisdiction was engaged in a process of shifting from welfare- to workfare-oriented social assistance policy, where work requirements were the norm and where the categories of social assistance recipients required to participate in work-incentive programs expanded to include single mothers with young children, especially those reluctant to attach themselves to a male partner. Ongoing developments in these two jurisdictions, however, continued to reflect their different histories and distinct contemporary trajectories. The erosion of AFDC and Food Stamps programs, plus a shift toward work incentives at the federal level since the early 1970s, contributed to an incremental but sustained transition in Wisconsin. In Ontario, work requirements were introduced only in the mid-1990s, following the election of a Conservative provincial government and the introduction at the federal level of the CHST.[17]

Wisconsin

Patterns of social assistance policy development in Wisconsin during the late 1990s were strikingly similar to policy restructuring activities occurring at the same time in Ontario. W-2, which dramatically altered public assistance provision in Wisconsin, went into effect before Ontario Works, however, and contained rules and requirements that were more explicitly gendered. Wisconsin could represent the outer limit (that is, the most extreme social experiment) where single mothers were concerned, since it imposed close scrutiny and monitoring of their behavior. Indeed, analysts routinely contend that the U.S. federal government followed the Wisconsin model in devising PRWORA and TANF.[18] Certainly, under W-2, Wisconsin's policy objectives and program design reflected and intensified the goals of PRWORA and TANF.

Wisconsin's central objective was to encourage all adults, including those with or expecting children, to leave social assistance and become "self-sufficient." Consistent with the TANF work requirements, W-2 also required all "employable" parents and custodians to engage in paid work, either once state authorities determined they were capable or after twenty-four months on assistance, whichever came sooner. As well, the program aimed to reduce the incidence of nonmarital births and to establish numerical goals for reducing the "illegitimacy ratio" in the state (see Gwendolyn Mink's discussion in chapter 6), a more explicit set of goals than prevailed in Ontario.

Wisconsin introduced a range of educational and "family planning" programs and a system of flat grants for families based on program participation, rather than on family size. The state eliminated additional payments for children "born more than ten months after the date that the W-2 participant was determined to be eligible for assistance or for a Wisconsin Works employment placement."[19] It also dictated that parents be subject to normal W-2 time limits if they have a child "more than ten months after the date the individual is first determined eligible for W-2 ... unless the birth was a result of sexual assault or incest," noting explicitly that its policy standard is "one of abstinence."[20] The state government's "employment focused family planning" and its enforcement of paternal responsibilities reinforced this standard. Only parents, the majority of whom were women, caring for a child under twelve weeks of age could receive social assistance benefits without participating in W-2, but women who had a child more than ten months after they went on assistance received no such exemption.

In addition to these measures, Wisconsin also introduced a Paternity Acknowledgment Through Hospitals (PATH) initiative. Through this program, the state used TANF funds for hospital-based paternity establishment, "for the purposes of coordinating and consolidating efforts to procure child support from non-custodial parents, and to provoke co-responsibility for the child."[21] The PATH program provided a $20 financial incentive to hospitals that persuaded mothers receiving public assistance to voluntarily establish paternity within sixty days of a child's birth. The hospital received the financial incentive only if the appropriate form was filed with the vital records office; this form became enforceable as a legal judgment that provided "conclusive determination of paternity."[22] In addition to PATH, Wisconsin provided for the authorization of genetic tests for paternity establishment.[23]

The state also received permission from the federal government to conduct a "parental responsibility pilot." This project would penalize more harshly single parents or dual-parent families that conceived a child while on public assistance and would place limits on state-administered earned-income supplements for these individuals.[24] As an extension of the child exclusion, or "family cap," rules examined by Gwendolyn Mink in chapter 6, this pilot project would further penalize women who conceived a child while on assistance.

Reflecting federal legislation passed in 1996, Wisconsin enforced a five-year lifetime limit on welfare. It offered a few exceptions for the disabled, people with severe limitations to employment, people needed in the home to care for a disabled family member, and people prevented from obtaining employment because local labor market conditions precluded reasonable job opportunities.[25] Wisconsin also set a twenty-four-month time limit on subsidized employment positions and denied public assistance to individuals who refused three times to participate in W-2.[26]

In design terms, W-2 was composed of two overarching streams, each encompassing various substreams that program architects viewed as part of an employment ladder.[27] Three parties were involved in the delivery of the program and charged with the task of moving social assistance recipients up the ladder: the financial and employment planner (who replaced the social service worker), the public assistance recipient, and the delivery agent or agency. The Department of Workforce Development in the state contracted out the delivery of W-2 programs, using a system of competitive bidding and payment based on performance.[28] As well, an employability plan was mandated, prefiguring Ontario Works' participation agreement.

The first stream of W-2 was unsubsidized employment. It formed the highest and most desirable component of W-2. Individuals deemed eligible for unsubsidized employment were offered vocational guidance, assistance with job survival and retention skills, and help with résumé-writing. First-stream participants were then often "matched with employers" who needed workers.

The second stream of W-2 was subsidized employment and work training. This stream was designed for participants who were unsuccessful in attempting to find jobs and were deemed unprepared for unsubsidized placement. Under subsidized placement, the applicant might be offered a trial job, meaning subsidized work-training placements intended to encourage employers to give permanent opportunities to participants "who appear to be job ready [but] have a weak work history."[29] In the trial jobs program, the W-2 agency entered into a contract with the employer and paid the employer a subsidy of about $300 per month, with the expectation that if the W-2 participant performed satisfactorily, the employer would offer that participant a permanent job.[30]

In contrast to trial jobs, the community service work stream under W-2 was designated for individuals who were not seen as ready for regular employment, especially where attempts to place the participant in an unsubsidized job were unsuccessful. This stream was intended to provide participants with opportunities to develop or improve work habits and skills perceived to be necessary to succeed in a work environment.[31] Participants in community service jobs were expected to work forty hours per week.[32] Wisconsin's monthly community service job benefit in 2000 was $673; this payment was reduced by $5.15 for every hour that the participant failed, without a legitimate reason, to participate in assigned activities.

A third option, W-2T, was a work-training placement for those deemed to have multiple barriers to employment. It was designed for assistance recipients who were unable to participate successfully in one of the other W-2 work-training placements or unsubsidized employment schemes because of alcohol or drug abuse, disability, or the need to remain at home to care for a disabled family member.

Ontario

Strong similarities exist between Wisconsin and Ontario, but the pace of change in social assistance policy was more rapid in the latter, even though its workfare regime was somewhat less advanced. Dramatic changes began in Ontario after 1995, with alterations to the General Welfare Assistance Act (1958) permitting the introduction of mandatory work requirements. Work requirements were formalized in 1998 when the Ontario Works Act (1997), a subset of the Social Assistance Reform Act (1997), replaced the Family Benefits Act (1967) and the General Welfare Assistance Act. Once the federal government ended the Canada Assistance Plan, particularly its provision that "no person shall be denied assistance because he refuses or has refused to take part in any work activity project," Ontario was able to initiate Canada's first mandatory welfare-to-work program through Ontario Works.[33]

New sets of policy objectives and social assistance programs emerged under the Ontario Works Act. Mirroring legislation in the United States, this act set out to "recognize individual responsibility" and "promote self-reliance through employment."[34] To this end, the Ontario Ministry of Community and Social Services introduced six changes designed to foster "self-sufficiency." The ministry as of 1998 included sole-support parents among those who were subject to mandatory work requirements, introduced new measures to reduce fraud, crafted improved delivery and monitoring systems, implemented new mandatory services for children, and instituted measures designed to limit social assistance recipients' ability to own their own homes.[35] Also mirroring W-2, the Ontario legislation "aims to provide temporary financial assistance to those in need while they satisfy obligations to become and stay employed."[36]

The conservative "family values" posture underpinning Ontario social assistance policies was apparent in decisions to reintroduce the cohabitation, or "man-in-the-house," rule, which allowed municipalities to deny social assistance recipients access to benefits if they were deemed to be in a "co-residency" situation with a member of the opposite sex.[37] To determine co-residency, the municipality must consider the financial relations between the parties, familial relations, and social relations in the household—but not sexual factors. If co-residency is established and if the spouse of the applicant is capable of supporting the applicant financially, then assistance is denied.[38] Although this provision was challenged with varying degrees of success,[39] the provincial government justified it on the basis that "couples who live together and have a spousal relationship should be treated the same as married couples when they apply for welfare."[40] Ironically, in imposing this rule, the Ontario Conservative government introduced a different definition of common-law marriage for low-income women than for those ineligible for (or not seeking) social assistance. In the former case, common-law assumptions and responsibilities were made as soon as cohabitation took place, while in the latter, they were made only after three years.

Another measure designed to encourage nuclear family formation and to end state support of women was the Ontario provision allowing the superintendent of welfare to pursue an independent child support application on behalf of the state.[41] The goal of this policy was to find an individual to support the single mother (ideally, a former spouse or partner) and ensure that he fulfilled his financial obligations, regardless of whether the mother chose to pursue support. Ontario's elimination of the $37 per month nutritional supplement for single mothers was a related measure that suggested the Conservative government viewed pregnancy as appropriate only for some women (that is, for women not on social assistance) and in specific contexts (nuclear families).[42] Each of these regulations was allowable under the terms of the 1996 CHST, but, more strikingly, each reflected the terms of the U.S. PRWORA, which explicitly constructed marriage and waged work as the primary (either/or) routes to self-sufficiency for single mothers.

In keeping with the ultimate objective of reducing women's dependence on the state, the provincial requirement that single mothers of children over 3.8 years of age participate in an Ontario Works program symbolized the meeting point of the conservative "family values" and neoliberal tenets of Ontario's social assistance regime. The provincial government saw mandatory work requirements for sole-support parents as "one of the most effective ways of breaking the cycle of dependency that can be so depressingly familiar: Grow up on welfare, live on welfare."[43] Crafted as a deterrent designed to prevent mothers from exiting spousal relationships, but less severe than its counterpart in Wisconsin, this requirement made a spousal relationship the only potential context in which mothers could "choose" to care for their own children indefinitely. At the same time, it was consistent with neoliberal policies mandating labor force participation when family and community supports fell short.

Legislative and regulatory changes in Ontario were accompanied by changes in social assistance delivery that introduced a harsher and more punitive regime. Through the Social Assistance Reform Act (SARA), Ontario Works conferred a more onerous set of obligations on social assistance recipients and instituted a lengthier application procedure for the receipt of benefits. Under this program, municipalities were permitted to establish a system of fingerprinting applicants and could require them to agree to participate in Ontario Works programs by signing application forms and consent forms before their claims were processed. In Ontario, Conservative social assistance legislation replaced the welfare appeal board with a small tribunal that had reduced scope. It also established a framework for the privatization of social assistance services to an extent that was not possible in the past.

Finally, Ontario developed a three-tiered set of social assistance programs, ranging from "pure workfare" (i.e., direct unpaid work in exchange for welfare) to "new style" workfare initiatives where most social assistance recipients must engage in training, trial jobs, and/or job searches to receive benefits.[44] Across these three tiers, which resembled Wisconsin's employment ladder, social assistance recipients were required to engage in a broad set of work-related activities, ranging from training, job seeking, schooling, and community work to paid and unpaid work in the private and public sectors. Based on their compliance with Ontario Works, recipients received direct or indirect income transfers from the provincial government.

The bottom tier of programs in Ontario Works involved community participation. Strikingly reminiscent of W-2's subsidized community-based jobs, this set of programs entailed the direct exchange of unpaid work for social assistance benefits from the government. Under existing guidelines, social assistance recipients must work for up to seventy hours per month in either a project created by the municipality or a nonprofit institution or organization. The second-tier programs offered "employment supports," which included basic education (i.e., upgrading to the maximum of a high school diploma) or job skills training in exchange for benefits and basic assistance with job searches. In general, employment support programs targeted those who faced significant barriers to labor market entry, frequently related to illiteracy or a lack of formal education, and thus resembled W-2T in Wisconsin.

Finally, the top tier of programs involved employment placement. This set of programs dealt with "employable" recipients, who were first prepared for private sector unsubsidized jobs and, subsequently, placed into available jobs, as was common in W-2's unsubsidized employment stream. Ontario guidelines for employment placement programs encouraged municipal social assistance departments to engage private sector delivery agents, such as private employment agencies, to place recipients in employment. Under this set of programs, delivery agents were rewarded on a performance basis.[45]

Conservative "Family Values" Meet Neoliberal Imperatives

In Wisconsin and Ontario, the significance of policies designed to shift single mothers' dependency from the state to the family went beyond efforts to institutionalize the nuclear family form. Not only did policies familialize single mothers' dependency, thereby undercutting poor women's access to full social citizenship as individuals, but they also augmented the state's control over social reproduction and reinforced the gender division of labor by failing to acknowledge the value of care work.[46] If single mothers were unable or unwilling to play a highly privatized (and undervalued) role in social reproduction, then they faced harsh penalties. When "marriage" was not an option, gender-neutral, neoliberal goals of "self-sufficiency" and "personal responsibility," which treated single mothers as "worker-citizens," replaced the principle of subsidiarity. In policy design and delivery, mandatory work for welfare became a fallback position when families failed.[47]

Once children reached a certain age in Wisconsin and Ontario, single mothers had to participate in one of three general types of workfare programs: community placement, job training, or employment placement (subsidized and unsubsidized).[48] Given this requirement, many questions arise. What types of opportunities do these programs offer for single mothers? Do they offer genuine economic independence, meaning a source of subsistence independent of the state and "the family?" How would single mothers' participation in W-2 or Ontario Works affect their social citizenship rights and entitlements as labor force participants? What are the effects of these programs on the gendered organization of the labor market?

Since W-2 and Ontario Works remain relatively new programs, their effects are not well documented. Yet the limitations of mandatory work-for-welfare programs for single mothers extend to the type of training provided. There was little evidence that the training streams in W-2 or Ontario Works offered genuine training or skills upgrading. Rather, in some cases, evidence suggested that the type of training provided amounted to socializing workers (women and men) to accept precarious employment. For example, flowing from TANF measures that restricted educational opportunities and limited allowable child-care expenses, Wisconsin's W-2 program excluded college training as a legitimate source of job preparation for low-income single mothers.[49] Instead, programs "trained" or streamed women into low-wage jobs, making genuine self-sufficiency at a decent standard of living a highly improbable outcome of work requirements.

Similarly, reflecting the Ontario government's explicit goal of finding the shortest route to paid employment and limiting education options to a high school diploma maximum, one municipality set up a program called Workfirst to place workers through temporary help agencies. The training component of the employment placement stream involved an orientation designed to acquaint participants with the "new" world of work, where employment relations are insecure, and to provide instruction on "dressing appropriately," interview skills, and time management, rather than on meaningful education or training.[50]

This type of employment placement program was designed to stream female social assistance recipients into low-end clerical and light industrial jobs. Restrictions on training, as well as the funneling of women into caregiving occupations in the market, made both the top rung of the employment ladder in Wisconsin and the third stream of Ontario Works virtually inaccessible to single mothers. Combined with a lack of accessible quality child care, these restrictions increased the likelihood that women would be placed in low-wage, low-skilled jobs with limited opportunities for advancement.[51]

In Wisconsin, a shortage of child-care provision triggered a notable trend. Since finding, securing, and keeping child care was key to maintaining employment, W-2 agencies encouraged many single mothers, especially social assistance recipients who were marginally employable or who reached the time limits in various programs, to become child-care providers through the market. In a study of low-income parents in Wisconsin, Diane Michalski

Turner observed that "the W-2 agency, in its eagerness to encourage everyone who could work to work, pushed them into becoming child-care providers" for two reasons: first, "these persons could meet the demand for child-care providers"; and, second, child-care provision was a viable employment option for "individuals [especially single mothers] who could not find other employment."[52]

Turner also found that W-2 staff expedited single mothers' registration as child-care providers by shortening the training program and modifying certification regulations. For the W-2 participant who required child care and who was engaged in training, subsidized or unsubsidized work, or a trial job, one consequence of this informal policy was a relatively unregulated child-care environment, in which the children of W-2 participants received care from providers who could not obtain employment in other sectors. Turner's study also found that these child-care providers frequently canceled their child-care services because they were in poor health. As a result, 55 of the 74 respondents in her study reported that they were terminated from or quit W-2 programs because of difficulties with child care.

Clearly, the movement toward channeling single mothers into child-care provision reflected the lack of meaningful employment options for single mothers under W-2 and the sex segregation that such programs perpetuated in the labor market. In practice, W-2 required single mothers to perform caregiving work for the children of other W-2 participants, effectively denying single mothers the opportunity to withdraw from the labor market to "care" for their own children and entrenching existing gender divisions so that women still remained responsible for care. These same types of problems were a genuine possibility in Ontario, given increased provincial autonomy under the terms of SUFA, the well-publicized shortage of subsidized child-care spaces, and the provincial government's endorsement of informal caregiving.[53]

In both Wisconsin and Ontario, the neoliberal tenets of mandatory work-for-welfare programs adopted the language of gender neutrality, but were unlikely to result in anything approximating substantive equality in the labor market or the domestic sphere. Instead, as earlier discussions of care politics by

Jane Jenson and Gwendolyn Mink would predict, they reinforced the conservative aim of refamilialization. Despite using slogans like "making work pay" to usher in work requirements, politicians could offer little convincing evidence that the type of waged work provided under W-2 or Ontario Works actually "pays" for the single mother. Not only were poor women denied the choice of caring for their own children in the private sphere and receiving state assistance and full social citizenship rights as mothers, but they were also denied genuine equality in labor market access and substance. Therefore, the combination of conservative policies rooted in "family values" discourse and neoliberal provisions embedded in these social assistance regimes reinforced the claim that women's roles in social reproduction were intricately intertwined with their subordinate location in the labor market. For this reason, alternative models aimed at achieving full social citizenship for the single mother need to recognize that, as it stands, she faces an impossible "choice" in jurisdictions like Wisconsin and Ontario: either reprivatization, refamilialization, and dependence on a man, rather than on the state, or else continued relegation to the bottom of the labor market, where even worker-citizenship is tenuous.

Care Allowances and Other Alternative Policies

Child-care shortages and the nature of welfare-to-work programs under W-2 and Ontario Works, which reinforce labor force segregation by sex, could prompt Wisconsin and Ontario to pay women for the work they perform in their "natural" role in social reproduction. One remedy for the apparent shortage of "care" in both settings might be to allow single mothers the choice to care for their children full time in the private sphere if no alternative support were available—that is, where no spouse was present or accountable.

In the context of W-2 and Ontario Works, recognizing caregiving could involve adding a caregiver stream—or some version of a care allowance—to existing program streams. Offering a care allowance would thus supplement training, pre-employment, and employment programs that Wisconsin and Ontario now mandate, a policy alternative that some feminists (including Gwendolyn Mink in chapter 6) support in principle and one that is worthy of serious scrutiny. Its very compatibility with conservative "family values" discourse and with neoliberal ideas underpinning both workfare regimes, however, makes the care allowance proposal particularly suspect.

Policies designed to recognize and value the socially necessary work of caregiving include the establishment of care allowances (described previously with reference to West European systems by Selma Sevenhuijsen in chapter 1 and Jane Jenson in chapter 3), as well as paid employment leaves and policies facilitating the collectivization of child care. In arguing that the welfare state is not simply a system of redistribution, but also a set of ideas about society, family, state, and market, feminist scholars have related a wide array of welfare state programs (including social assistance) to social reproduction. Their work reveals the critical link between state social provision and caregiving and highlights the need for a nuanced and gender-sensitive understanding of what welfare state theorists term *decommodification*, or freedom from reliance on labor markets.[54]

Women's complex roles in the welfare state,[55] particularly their central role in various facets of social reproduction, led many feminist scholars to examine what Carole Pateman identifies as "Wollstonecraft's dilemma." This refers to the dilemma over whether the claims women make on the state should be based on notions of equality or difference.[56] To overcome this dilemma, Pateman advocated a redefinition of work (both paid and unpaid) that would result in a new form of female citizenship, designed partly to raise the status of social reproduction. Taking a similar course, other feminist scholars who supported policies aimed at legitimizing women's caregiving activities did so on the basis of "difference" claims that reflected a discomfort with casting decommodification as the central objective of social provision. Their approach suggested that the capacity to earn a wage was central to women's full social citizenship.

According to this part of the feminist literature, measures such as care allowances and gender-specific paid leaves aim to equalize women's and men's citizenship entitlements, by introducing an alternative route to full social citizenship. Rather than using the traditional model of worker-citizenship, where the welfare state was organized on an occupational basis and where the full social citizen was assumed to be a full-time, full-year, paid employed male, feminists proposed a range of measures that permitted women (and men who chose to care) to gain access to social citizenship through their caregiving activities. The policies endorsed in feminist scholarship and applied most fully to the case of single mothers were of three general types: care allowances, paid leaves from employment, and collectivized caregiving.

Growing numbers of scholars support the introduction of care allowances for single mothers, as well as for people who care for the elderly, as one way to give women independent access to subsistence and hence a broader set of social citizenship rights. A leading proponent of such allowances for single mothers is Gwendolyn Mink, the author of chapter 6 in this volume, who advocates their introduction in order to "restore mothers' constitutional rights—to not marry, to bear children, and to parent alone, even if they are poor."[57] For Mink, care allowances would "promote occupational freedom, by rewarding work even when work cannot be exchanged for wages. So redefined, welfare would become a sign not of dependency but of independence, a means not to moral regulation but to social and political justice."[58]

Mink's vision is one in which poor single mothers, who are disproportionately African-American in the United States, could choose to care for their own children, rather than to accept low-wage, dead-end jobs. The latter often involve caring for the children of others and perpetuate a highly racialized gender division of labor. Mink does not view care allowances as a panacea, but rather as an intervention designed to offset a negative set of policies. Her notion is consistent with the ideas of Carole Pateman in several respects, primarily because it involves revaluing unpaid work and caregiving as the basis for a new form of female citizenship.[59]

Another model for recognizing and rewarding care involves the provision of paid leaves from employment. In some national contexts where they are the norm, paid parental leaves, and even general family leaves, are almost exclusively reserved for women, despite the presence of a male partner.[60] The United States, which has provided unpaid leave at the national level since 1993, is a case in point. In other jurisdictions, paid leave policies are usually gender-neutral on their face and offer women and men access to paid leaves to fulfill family obligations on the basis of their status as worker-citizens. In practice, however, many of these policies have gender-specific effects, since to gain the right to state support for dependent children, *potential mothers must first be waged workers*.

Sweden's paid leave policies provide an interesting and instructive example of this type of measure. In the Swedish case, women's entitlements to welfare and family policies changed drastically after the early 1970s. According to Lewis and Astrom, the state shifted "away from the provision of benefits to them as mothers toward benefits that they [women] draw by virtue of their labour market status"[61] The effects of this transition were highly contradictory for women. Women had to participate in the paid labor force in order to obtain generous family leaves that actively encourage them to care for young children in the private sphere. Moreover, even though all Swedish women were encouraged to do paid work, once they became mothers (and therefore became entitled to generous family leaves), many found it difficult to access segments of the labor market that were inhospitable to workers with family responsibilities.

Parallel with arguments presented by Sevenhuijsen and Jenson in earlier chapters, the practical consequences of this confluence of policies remain far from trivial: the great majority of Swedish women work in the public sector, performing work formerly done unpaid by women in the home, and a sizable percentage work part time in low-status service jobs in order to juggle other demands on their time.[62] Sex segregation permeates the labor market, on the one hand, while women continue to do a disproportionate amount of unpaid work, on the other.[63]

A third group of measures designed to recognize the centrality of care in the welfare state attempts to lessen the familial responsibilities of mothers and other kin and to open up vocational opportunities for them. Most gender-neutral in its aims, this model involves the collectivization of caregiving through, for example, public child-care facilities.⁶⁴ Like paid leave policies, collectivized caregiving is often associated with the view that all citizens should be workers; as a result, daycare is frequently constructed as a "child minding service for working parents." However, some proponents of this approach argue that public collective child care is a socially responsible and appropriate way to care for children, since it plays a socialization function, regardless of the centrality of waged work in the broader society.⁶⁵ If applied to single-mother households, this type of measure would make caregiving a collective and public responsibility, managed by the state as one of its central welfare functions.

Each of these strategies has its merits. Valuing caregiving through care allowances can contribute to making "care" a more central dimension of social citizenship. At a practical level, it could give single mothers independent access to social rights, entitlements, and a basic standard of living if they chose to care for their own children. These are very worthy aims, particularly in North American jurisdictions where the racialized gender division of labor has prevented many women from looking after their own children full time and instead has forced them to engage in other forms of low-wage work.⁶⁶

Policies connected with leaves, too, have several strengths, since they enable mothers to recover from the strains of procreation and allow time for breastfeeding and bonding between mother and child. Similarly, remedying obstacles to women's full social citizenship through the provision of child care that is affordable, collective, accessible, and publicly administered has been a central demand of the modern women's movement since its inception. For single mothers in particular, this alternative has the advantage of making the "choice" between labor force participation and waged work (or some combination of the two options) more genuine.

The advantages of measures designed to valorize women's complex caregiving roles in the welfare state are important to emphasize. However, each alternative has serious limitations if it is adopted as the primary route toward gender equality and access to social citizenship rights for women. The central shortcomings of all these measures are threefold. First, all continue to allow men to choose not to care. Even in cases where strong incentives exist for men to care, as in Norway and increasingly Sweden, their caregiving responsibilities are limited.

Second, as Selma Sevenhuijsen and Jane Jenson note in chapters 1 and 3, these measures have the potential to reinforce sex segregation in the labor market and rigid divisions of labor in the domestic sphere. Following on Dionne Bensonsmith's arguments in chapter 2, valuing caregiving can have particularly perverse effects in racially divided societies. None of these policies alters the common presumption that it is primarily women who will engage in service or caregiving work, whether paid or unpaid. Third, each alternative brackets inequities generated by the gendered organization (or segmentation) of the labor market. As we know from the Swedish case, this is a grave error because women still predominate in caregiving occupations, even when various facets of social reproduction have been collectivized.[67] Hence, it is important to highlight the limitations of strategies focused exclusively on valuing care, especially when they are advanced on their own or when feminist scholars are forced to wield them defensively.

As a response to the introduction of workfare-oriented social assistance policies in Wisconsin and Ontario, proposals that the state pay for care of one's own children (or the children of women in like situations) are easily manipulated by interests seeking to reprivatize social reproduction and relegate women to the domestic sphere. Under the regimes in question, where mandatory work for welfare is becoming the norm, these policies are a recipe for intensified income and occupational segregation by sex—since they neither address the gendered organization of the labor market nor make men care—and for continued poverty among single mothers.

Conclusion

Several variations on these alternative policy options could be introduced under a caregiver stream in W-2 and Ontario Works. One example is some form of paid leave policy for single mothers who become pregnant while participating in W-2 or Ontario Works, resembling parental leave policies available to regular employees in the United States and Canada. Indeed, creating a fourth caregiver stream for social assistance provision is a logical extension of prevailing attempts under both workfare regimes to legitimize women's role in social reproduction. In the Canadian context, this stream would coincide with the efforts of various groups to highlight women's disproportionate share of unpaid work and, by extension, to defend single mothers' exemption from mandatory work-for-welfare programs.[68] These policy and programmatic alternatives, no doubt, have growing purchase among feminist scholars who advocate greater "choice" for women in the short and medium term in both jurisdictions.

Under these two workfare regimes, however, the limitations of a caregiver stream are striking. In countries where they do exist, care-oriented strategies designed to secure genuine choice for single mothers (but not necessarily gender equality) are Band-Aid or temporary measures, rather than transformative solutions that reconfigure gendered labor market and domestic situations. In the case of care allowances, as Jane Jenson demonstrates in chapter 3, empirical evidence suggests that they generally offer relatively low levels of remuneration for caregiving work, at best, and nominal cash honorariums, at worst.

Leave policies, too, not only retain the gendered status quo where caregiving is concerned, but can potentially contribute to reprivatizing caregiving and entrenching sex-based divisions of labor in the domestic sphere. Conditions related to labor force participation are also usually attached to the receipt of such benefits. That these policies fail to alter the gendered structure of social reproduction and, as numerous scholars emphasize, do little to "make men care," is highly problematic. Extensive leave policies also have the potential to perpetuate sex segregation by encouraging flexible employment policies in female-dominated areas of the labor market, leaving male-dominated domains virtually untouched by the daily and intergenerational requirements of caregiving. They thus threaten to reinforce patterns of labor force participation, where women dominate in jobs that reflect tasks conventionally associated with social reproduction, and where they are confined to atypical and contingent employment relationships because these are the only employment arrangements that enable them to accommodate family responsibilities.

Although it holds some potential from a gender-equality perspective, even the provision of accessible public child care is insufficient, if it is the only means used to redress women's unequal social citizenship in a context of sharp labor force segmentation by sex and the introduction of workfare. Adopting this last alternative is especially problematic if public provision is justified on the basis that welfare states are primarily "about work and workers," as Jane Jenson notes, and if women continue to perform the bulk of caregiving work in the labor market (at low wages) and the domestic sphere (at low or no wages).[69] Posed in these terms, universal public child care provides little impetus for men to become child-care workers in the market, nor does it compel men to engage in unpaid caregiving activities at home.

If a fourth caregiver stream, composed of care allowances for single mothers (or even some other mix of paid leave policies, care allowances, and publicly accessible child care), were to be introduced in Wisconsin and Ontario, it would probably not contribute to fundamental gender equality outcomes. Without altering the direction of social assistance provision and without the introduction of measures designed to reorganize (and hence desegregate) the labor market, care allowances in particular would further entrench a division of labor in which low-income women are expected to care for dependent children and adults.

Given these limits, two new directions for further research are worth exploring. In pursuing them, the aim should *not* be to abandon creative alternatives designed to elevate care in search of greater equality for single mothers on social assistance. Instead, we need to improve the alternatives and develop complementary measures aimed at achieving gender equality inside the labor market.

First, at a conceptual level, scholars need to abandon the work/care dichotomy that prevails in much of the contemporary literature on the welfare state. As Sevenhuijsen and Jenson argue in earlier chapters, this approach obscures the strong and necessary relationship between the supply and demand sides of the labor market, encompassing social reproduction and production. Rather than using dichotomous thinking, we would be better off addressing "questions of who cares, who pays, and where care is provided," in order to broaden our understanding of the welfare/work nexus and its effects on single mothers.[70] Pursued as a long-term strategy, efforts to rethink the welfare state in this way would prompt an end to workfare altogether and could contribute to a genuinely alternative vision of gender justice. As a short-term strategy, it would necessitate immediate changes in policy design and delivery.

Second, since waged labor is the primary source of subsistence for citizens in contemporary liberal welfare states, we need to pursue a concrete set of short-term measures rooted in ideals of gender equality and designed to both eliminate labor market segmentation by sex and legitimize a "universal caregiver model."[71] Combining supply and demand-side measures would enable women to choose *not* to care in the labor market, and would permit them to place greater restrictions on caregiving activities in the domestic sphere. At the same time, it would encourage men to do more caring in both spheres. Ideally, the mix would include active labor market policies to promote meaningful employment and other strategies to revalue a range of caring or caregiving professions. The recognition and expectation that caregiving responsibilities are universal (and shared by states and citizens) would lie at the root of each set of policies.

These two directions for further investigation do not constitute a research program, nor are they completely new, since feminist scholars have in the past raised many related questions and issues. However, they are necessary supplements to the narrow set of prevailing alternatives aimed at improving the situation of single mothers on social assistance. Developments in social assistance policy in Wisconsin and Ontario, which amount to the introduction of welfare-to-work policies rooted in conservative "family values" and neoliberal ideas, highlight the need for more innovative approaches and new research trajectories in the age of workfare.

Notes

The author wishes to thank the Canada Research Chair program and the Social Sciences and Humanities Research Council of Canada for their financial assistance and Maureen Baker, Sylvia Bashevkin, Sandra

Burt, Gerald Kernerman, Rianne Mahon, Kim McIntyre, Gwendolyn Mink, Ann Shola Orloff, and Iris Marion Young for their constructive comments. All monetary amounts cited in this chapter are reported in the currency of the country in question.

1. See Barbara Hobson, "No Exit, No Voice: Women's Economic Dependency and the Welfare State," *Acta Sociologica* 33 (1990): 235–50; Barbara Hobson, "Solo Mothers, Social Policy Regimes, and the Logics of Gender," in *Gendering Welfare States*, ed. Diane Sainsbury (London: Sage, 1994), 170–87; Arnlaug Leira, *Welfare States and Working Mothers: The Scandinavian Experience* (Cambridge: Cambridge University Press, 1992); and Jane Lewis, "Gender and the Development of Welfare Regimes," *Journal of European Social Policy* 2 (1992): 159–73.
2. See Maureen Baker and David Tippin, *Poverty, Social Assistance, and the Employability of Mothers* (Toronto: University of Toronto Press, 1999); Sylvia Bashevkin, "Rethinking Retrenchment: North American Social Policy during the Early Clinton and Chrétien years," *Canadian Journal of Political Science* 33 (2000): 7–36; and Gwendolyn Mink, *Welfare's End* (Ithaca, N.Y.: Cornell University Press, 1998).
3. See Patricia Evans and Gerda Wekerle, eds., *Women and the Canadian Welfare State* (Toronto: University of Toronto Press, 1997); Bridgette Kitchen, "'Common Sense': Assaults on Families," in *Open for Business, Closed to People*, ed. D. Ralph, A. Regimbald, and N. St. Amand (Halifax: Fernwood, 1997), 103–12; and Katherine Rhoades and Anne Statham, eds., *Speaking Out: Women, Poverty, and Public Policy* (Madison: University of Wisconsin System Women's Studies Librarian, 1999).
4. In this chapter, the phrase "conservative 'family values'" refers to a set of ideas about family and society that assumes women's place is in the domestic sphere, marriage is the proper domain in which to raise children, and the nuclear family is the foundational unit in advanced industrial societies. It is used to help identify the origins of a particular set of political practices and public policies. For further discussion of "conservative 'family values'" and "family politics," see Meg Luxton and Leah F. Vosko, "Where Women's Efforts Count: The 1996 Census Campaign and 'Family Politics' in Canada," *Studies in Political Economy* 56 (1998): 43–82.
5. The movement toward workfare in Wisconsin and Ontario, and its implications for the single mother, form the central focus of this chapter. Thus, the discussion of care allowances and other measures designed to recognize and value women's caregiving work, while a necessary and important endpoint for the ensuing analysis, remains preliminary.
6. Gerard Boychuk, *Patchworks of Purpose: The Development of Provincial Social Assistance Regimes in Canada* (Montreal: McGill-Queen's University Press, 1999).
7. Beginning in 1972, AFDC required all employable welfare recipients in the United States to participate in work incentive programs. However, the Omnibus Budget Reconciliation Act

(1981) and Family Support Act (1988) were instrumental in advancing a view of social assistance benefits as transitional to paid work for lone mothers.

8. Changes to AFDC included the introduction of work incentive programs in 1972, as well as a drift toward mandatory work requirements under the terms of the Reagan-era Omnibus Reconciliation Act (1981) and Family Support Act (1988).
9. See Mink, *Welfare's End*.
10. United States Congress, Personal Responsibility and Work Opportunity Reconciliation Act of 1996 (H.R. 3734), Title 1, pt. A.
11. Ibid., preamble.
12. Ibid., sec. 401 (a).
13. Nancy Fraser and Linda Gordon, "A Geneology of Dependency: Tracing a Keyword of the U.S. Welfare State," *Signs* 19 (1994): 309–36.
14. Gerard Boychuk, *Are Canadian and U.S. Social Assistance Policies Converging?* (Orono: University of Maine Canadian-American Center, 1997), 14.
15. Katherine Scott, *Women and the CHST: A Profile of Women Receiving Social Assistance in 1994* (Ottawa: Status of Women Canada, 1998), 17.
16. Given this rigid requirement, it is not surprising that some prominent feminists in the United States called for care allowances or guaranteed annual incomes to protect women's individual entitlements to social citizenship as mothers.
17. Interestingly, programs in Ontario closely resembled the immediate precursors to Wisconsin's W-2 welfare-to-work initiative, which were developed under first the U.S. federal waiver system and then the 1972 federal Work Incentive Program.
18. Michael Massing, "The End of Welfare?" *New York Review of Books* (October 7, 1999): 22.
19. Wisconsin Department of Workforce Development, *Wisconsin State Plan for Fiscal Year 1999-2000 for Administration of the Block Grant to States for Temporary Assistance for Needy Families* (July 22, 1999), 3.
20. Ibid., 2.
21. Ibid., 17.
22. Ibid.
23. State of Wisconsin, Public Assistance Act, chap. 49, sec. 49.225(2)(a), 1998.
24. Ibid.
25. These exceptions are important because they provide the state with a degree of flexibility in implementing W-2 and suggest that failure to find employment is not necessarily the result of an individual's lack of self-sufficiency or personal responsibility, but instead may result from labor market conditions.
26. See Wisconsin Department of Workforce Development, *Wisconsin State Plan*, 7. In order to encourage waged work, Wisconsin

created an extensive system of earned income tax credits. It also provided child-care subsidies to families whose income was less than 165 percent of the federal poverty line. Families remained eligible for this subsidy until their incomes reached 200 percent of the federal poverty line. See State of Wisconsin, Public Assistance Act, sec. 49.156.

27. In debates over Ontario Works, opposition members of the Ontario legislature referred explicitly to the Wisconsin model to highlight their concerns about the potential results of imposing mandatory work requirements. For example, on August 19, 1997, provincial opposition legislator Sandra Pupatello noted:

> Let me say that workfare is not new. It's not new to Ontario. It's not new to Canada. It has certainly been tried in many jurisdictions in North America, specifically in the United States. *Since we looked at other jurisdictions so carefully, why didn't we go further to ask these jurisdictions what kind of results they were seeing from bringing in workfare? I wanted to mention the Wisconsin model in particular, because now, after having introduced workfare some time ago, we're starting to see some significant results, and I might tell you it's not a pretty picture.* (Sandra Pupatello, as quoted in *Hansard* [Ontario legislative debates, August 19, 1997], emphasis added.)

Pupatello went on to describe what she saw as the results of W-2, which included a 25 percent increase in the numbers of people using homeless shelters in Milwaukee, a 14 percent increase in visits to food banks, and a 20 percent increase in visits to soup kitchens. By invoking the Wisconsin case, critics like Pupatello revealed an element of information-sharing among social assistance experts in the two jurisdictions.

28. The shift toward competitive bidding for public assistance delivery under the two overarching streams of W-2 signified a dramatic change in the administration of Wisconsin Works. Under AFDC, private entities were prohibited from determining eligibility or managing cases, and, as a result, public officials delivered programs. In 1994, Wisconsin introduced performance contracting for public assistance delivery; the state required centers to compete for the right to administer programs and linked W-2 agency compensation to performance. By introducing performance contracting, the state cut $10.25 million from its budget in the first two years of W-2. Public delivery agents still dominate in W-2, but a disproportionate number of private for-profit agents and faith-based, private nonprofit agencies operate in Wisconsin's largest cities. See David Dodenhoff, "Privatizing Welfare and Wisconsin: Ending Administrative Entitlement—W-2's Untold Story," *Wisconsin Policy Research Institute Report* 11, January 1998, 12–15.

29. Wisconsin Department of Workforce Development, *Wisconsin State Plan*, 9.

30. An individual could participate in a trial job for a maximum of three months and request a three-month extension if additional time were needed to assure job readiness. Individuals could participate at the trial job level for a maximum of twenty-four

months. In this stream of W-2, employers were expected to pay at least the minimum wage, as well as wages and benefits comparable to those received by regular employees in similarly classified positions.
31. Wisconsin Department of Workforce Development, *Wisconsin State Plan*, 9.
32. Individuals were also permitted to participate in the community service stream for no more than twenty-four months.
33. For the terms of the Canada Assistance Plan, see *Revised Statutes of Canada*, chap. C-1, pt. III, sec. 15(3), 1985.
34. See Ontario Works Act, *Revised Statutes of Ontario*, chap. 25, sec. 1 (1999).
35. Janet Ecker, as quoted in *Hansard* (Ontario legislative debates, August 19, 1997).
36. Ontario Works Act.
37. The cohabitation rule was first introduced by the Ontario Liberal government of David Peterson, under the General Welfare Assistance Act. As the result of a challenge related to the definition of "common-law spouses," this rule was modified and subsequently removed in 1987. The Conservative government elected in 1995 reintroduced cohabitation limits under the General Welfare Assistance Act and then included them under the Ontario Works Act. According to Bridgette Kitchen, "the foremost reason given by the [provincial] government for its reversal of the cohabitation rule is its concern with reducing the Ontario budget deficit." Kitchen argues that the provincial government expected to save about $45 million a year by reintroducing this measure. Notably, in its first three years of operation, the cohabitation rule meant that nearly 7,000 women lost their entitlements to social assistance benefits, twice as many as had been expected. See Kitchen, "'Common Sense,'" 110–11.
38. Ontario Ministry of Community and Social Services, "Directive No. 14: Determining Co-Residency," *Ontario Works: Making Welfare Work* (June 1, 1998).
39. In 1996, four women who had been classified as "spouses" challenged the constitutionality of Ontario's new cohabitation rule. These applicants sought an order declaring Regulation 409/95, sec. 2(3) 1(2), of the Family Benefits Act to be unconstitutional. Even though they had cohabitated with a member of the opposite sex for less than a year and welfare workers had advised them that they would not be disqualified from family benefits until they had cohabitated for a period of three years, these women were denied benefits. Notably, none of the men was a father of the complainants' children, but the welfare department made a presumption of dependence. A majority of judges dismissed the application, claiming that a challenge under the Canadian Charter of Rights and Freedoms was premature. Instead, they called on the Social Assistance Review Board of Ontario to undertake a review of this provision. One dissenting opinion was recorded among the judges who heard the case; J. Rosenberg concluded that the

cohabitation rule was in violation of sec. 15 of the Charter, since it set a different standard for determining common law marriage among social assistance recipients (one year) than among the rest of the population (three years). See *Faulkner et al. v. Ontario*, Dominion Law Reports, 4th ed., 140 (1997), 172. The Social Assistance Review Board in 1998 found that the definition of "spouse" used in new social assistance legislation did indeed violate the applicants' constitutional rights. However, because the Ontario government appealed the board's decision, the cohabitation rule and its definition of "spouse" still hold in the province.

40. Ontario Ministry of Community and Social Services, *News Release*, September 4, 1998.
41. Ontario Works Act, chap. 25, sec. 134, 13(1).
42. According to Premier Mike Harris, the provincial government rescinded the nutritional supplement for pregnant women on social assistance "so that those dollars don't go to beer, don't go to something else." Premier Mike Harris, as quoted in Daniel Girard and Patricia Orwen, "Harris Sorry for 'Beer' Crack: Remark Angers Pregnant Women Receiving Welfare," *Toronto Star* (February 17, 1998), A1, A32. This measure was comparable to the type of penalties confronted by poor pregnant women in Wisconsin.
43. Ecker, as quoted in *Hansard*, August 19, 1997.
44. See Ernie Lightman, "You Can Lead a Horse to Water, but ... : The Case against Workfare in Canada," in *Helping the Poor: A Qualified Case for "Workfare,"* ed. J. Richards et al. (Toronto: C. D. Howe Institute, 1995), 154.
45. For a discussion of the role of private sector delivery agents, see Leah F. Vosko, "Workfare Temporaries: Workfare and the Rise of the Temporary Employment Relationship in Ontario," *Canadian Review of Social Policy* 42 (1998): 55–80.
46. I am grateful to Iris Young for convincing me of the importance of this last point.
47. Power resource theorists conventionally focus on citizens' social welfare when markets fail, highlighting the necessity of state intervention in the economy. See Gøsta Esping-Andersen, *Social Foundations of Postindustrial Economies* (Oxford: Oxford University Press, 1999). Yet in the absence of state intervention, when governments are willing to regulate social reproduction but not intervene directly, the pressing question is, What are women's options—specifically, single mothers' options—when families fail?
48. In Wisconsin, single mothers, like other social assistance recipients, can proceed through these three streams in consecutive steps.
49. See Sarah Harder, "W-2 Welfare Reforms: Undoing the Wisconsin Idea?" in *Speaking Out*, ed. Rhoades and Statham, 56–64.
50. For a detailed description of the Workfirst program, see Vosko, "Workfare Temporaries."

51. In Sweden, single mothers joined the labor force in significant numbers after the early 1980s. The Swedish labor market remains highly segregated (more so than in the United States and Canada), and women are disproportionately represented in nonstandard forms of employment. Women's wages are relatively high, however, since caregiving work is generally in the public sector. Thus, even with supply-side policies that support privatized caregiving activities through paid leaves, Swedish women continue to face barriers to full social citizenship. This situation highlights the importance of addressing obstacles confronted by women, both as labor force participants and as mothers or caregivers in the welfare state. See Jane Lewis and Gertrude Astrom, "Equality, Difference, and State Welfare: Labor Market and Family Policies in Sweden," *Feminist Studies* 18 (1992): 59–87; and Jane Lewis, "Gender and the Development of Welfare Regimes," *Journal of European Social Policy* 2 (1992): 159–73.

52. Diane Michalski Turner, "Stated and Unstated Needs: Low-Income Parents and Childcare," in *Speaking Out*, ed. Rhoades and Statham, 79.

53. Despite a growing recognition of child-care shortages in Ontario, limited documentation exists on the consequences of this shortage. See KPMG, "Ontario Works: Introduction and Summary," unpublished brief to the Ontario government, May 21, 1999; and Katherine Side, "Government Restraint and Limits to Economic Reciprocity in Women's Friendships," *Atlantis* 22 (1998): 5–15.

54. The question of whether decommodification is desirable for women is debated vigorously among feminists. Some argue that gendering social rights requires altering conventional views of decommodification, so that "the extent to which states guarantee women access to paid employment and services that enable them to balance home and work responsibilities" is taken into account (Ann Shola Orloff, "Gender and the Social Rights of Citizenship," *American Sociological Review* 58 [1993]: 303). Others, in contrast, argue that decommodification is central to achieving women's equality, but must be defined more broadly to include the state provision of care, including paid leave provisions or services that minimize tensions between paid and unpaid work for the working mother. As Rianne Mahon suggests, the redefined notion of decommodification involves "the extent to which states confront the *fictional* character of labour power as a commodity by supporting daily and intergenerational reproduction" (Rianne Mahon, "Childcare in Canada and Sweden: Policy and Politics," *Social Politics* 4 [1997]: 386). In critiquing various supply-side measures, especially care allowances, this chapter is informed by a parallel understanding of decommodification and its emancipatory potential for women, but recognizes the limits of conventional definitions of decommodification, as advanced by power resource theorists.

55. Beginning with the work of Elizabeth Wilson, feminists generally identified three dominant roles for women inside the welfare

state—executants, clients, and those charged with social reproduction—and emphasized that the contradictions and tensions raised by these overlapping roles necessitate creative interventions on the part of the state, organized labor, and other civil society groups. See Elizabeth Wilson, *Women and the Welfare State* (London: Tavistock, 1977). For pivotal Canadian works identifying the complex interplay among women's roles in the welfare state, see Caroline Andrew, "Women and the Welfare State," *Canadian Journal of Political Science* 17 (1984): 667–83; and Jane Jenson, "Gender and Reproduction, or, Babies and the State," *Studies in Political Economy* 20 (1986): 9–46.

56. Carole Pateman, "The Patriarchal Welfare State," in *Democracy and the Welfare State*, ed. Amy Gutman (Princeton: Princeton University Press, 1988): 231–60.

57. Mink, *Welfare's End*, 137.

58. Ibid.

59. Care allowances of the sort that Mink envisions already exist, to some degree, in Britain and Ireland. But prevailing schemes are not designed to further the ends that Mink seeks. In Britain, an invalid allowance for caregivers involves payments administered through the social security system. Initially, married women were excluded from this allowance. However, subject to an important court ruling, this policy changed in 1986. Under Britain's invalid allowance, no contract exists between the caregiver and the state that is designed to ensure that women carry out specific duties. Rather, monitoring is largely absent and the commodification of caregiving labor is limited. Partly as a result of this limited commodification, which rewards caregivers minimally, invalid allowances are very low, and women caregivers' public or private dependence is reduced but not eliminated. See Birte Sim, "Engendering Democracy: Social Citizenship and Political Participation for Women in Scandinavia," *Social Politics* 1 (1994): 4–31. In the feminist literature calling for the creation of care allowances for single mothers, debates focus on whether payments should come in direct exchange for specified work activities. See Clare Ungerson, "Social Politics and the Commodification of Care," *Social Politics* 4 (1997): 362–81; Jet Bussemaker, "Rationales of Care in Contemporary Welfare States: The Case of Childcare in the Netherlands," *Social Politics* 5 (1998): 70–96; and Arnlaug Leira, "Caring as a Social Right: The Case for Childcare and Daddy Leave," *Social Politics* 5 (1998): 362–78.

60. See Bussemaker, "Rationales of Care"; and Leira, "Caring as a Social Right."

61. See Lewis and Astrom, "Equality, Difference, and State Welfare," 59. For additional work that supports this conclusion, see Rianne Mahon, "'Both Wage Earner and Mother':Women's Organizing and Childcare Policy in Sweden and Canada," in *Women's Organizing and Public Policy in Canada and Sweden*, ed. Linda Briskin and Mona Eliasson (Montreal: McGill-Queen's University Press, 1999), 238–79.

62. Sweden's family leave system is more robust than that of either Canada or the United States; see Mahon, "Childcare in Canada and Sweden." Unemployment insurance schemes in Canada have been reformed since the Mulroney years and provide paid maternity leave to an ever narrower category of eligible women workers; see Leah F. Vosko, "Irregular Workers, New Involuntary Social Exiles: Women and UI Reform," in *Remaking Canadian Social Policy: Social Security in the Late 1990s*, ed. Jane Pulkingham and Gordon Turnowetsky (Toronto: Fernwood, 1996), 256-72.
63. One variation on prevailing paid leave policies also merits attention. In some social democratic welfare states, women and men are required or encouraged to share paid parental leaves. Norway has begun to experiment with a policy where *only* men can take a specified portion of leave to care for their infant children, and Sweden is following suit. This program is unique, in that it actively encourages men to "care"; if men do not take up a given portion of paid caregiving leave for children, this portion of the parental leave is lost completely. Since it actively seeks to induce greater gender equity in child care from infancy, this policy is a response to the gendered effects of paid leave policies, where men's take-up rate is very low. See Bussemaker, "Rationales of Care"; and Leira, "Caring as a Social Right."
64. Elder-care facilities and long-term care facilities for the disabled and the sick are consistent with this model.
65. See Martha Friendly, *Childcare Policy in Canada: Putting the Pieces Together* (Toronto: Addison-Wesley, 1994); and Luxton and Vosko, "Where Women's Efforts Count." For a review of the range of views held by American feminists on childcare over the course of the twentieth century, see Sonya Michel, *Children's Interests, Mothers' Rights* (New Haven: Yale University Press, 1999).
66. The same trend is true with respect to foreign domestic workers in Canada. See Sedef Arat-Koc, "'Importing Housewives': Non-citizen Domestic Workers and the Crisis of the Domestic Sphere in Canada," in *Through the Kitchen Window*, by Meg Luxton, Harriet Rosenberg, and Sedef Arat-Koc (Toronto: Garamond, 1990), 81-104.
67. In Sweden, "labor flexibility" policies that allow workers to fulfill family responsibilities are only available in certain segments of the labor market, notably female-dominated sectors. Therefore, women do not experience the benefits of a solidaristic wage policy because they are concentrated in a very limited number of female-dominated sectors of the economy. See Mahon, "Childcare in Canada and Sweden"; and Lewis and Astrom, "Equality, Difference, and State Welfare," 72-73.
68. Luxton and Vosko, "Where Women's Efforts Count." *Social Politics* 4(1997): 184.
69. Jane Jenson, "Gender and Welfare Regimes: Who Cares?"
70. Ibid., 187.
71. See Nancy Fraser, *Justice Interruptus* (London: Routledge, 1997), 59-62.

Contributors

Maureen Baker is a professor of sociology at the University of Auckland in New Zealand. She is the author of numerous articles and books, including *Canadian Family Policies: Cross-National Comparisons* (1995); *Poverty, Social Assistance, and the Employability of Mothers* (1999, with David Tippin); and *Families, Labour, and Love* (2001).

Sylvia Bashevkin is a professor of political science at the University of Toronto in Toronto, Ontario, Canada. She has published widely on Canadian and comparative politics and is the author of *Women on the Defensive: Living through Conservative Times* (1998) and *Welfare Hot Buttons: Women, Work, and Social Policy Reform* (2002).

Dionne Bensonsmith is a doctoral candidate in political science at Syracuse University in Syracuse, New York. Her chapter on the Moynihan Report is drawn from a larger dissertation project on welfare reform politics in the United States.

Jane Jenson holds a Tier I Canada Research Chair in political science at the Université de Montréal in Montreal, Quebec, Canada. She has contributed to many different areas of social science research, including electoral studies, political economy, social policy, and citizenship theory. She is the editor, with Mariette Sineau, of *Who Cares? Women's Work, Childcare, and Welfare State Redesign* (2001).

Gwendolyn Mink is a professor of government at Smith College in Northampton, Massachusetts. She is the author of many articles and books, including *The Wages of Motherhood* (1995), *Welfare's End* (1998), and *Hostile Environment* (2000), and the editor of *Whose Welfare?* (1999).

Selma Sevenhuijsen is a political theorist and professor in the ethics and politics of care at the University of Utrecht in the Netherlands. She has written extensively on women and the state, women and family law, and feminist political theory. Her most recent book is *Citizenship and the Ethics of Care: Feminist Considerations on Justice, Morality, and Politics* (1998), published by Routledge.

Leah F. Vosko holds a Tier II Canada Research Chair in political science at Atkinson College, York University in Toronto, Ontario, Canada. She is the author of *Temporary Work: The Gendered Rise of a Precarious Employment Relationship* (2000).

Index

abortion rates, 3, 153
abstinence education, 153–54, 174
Adoption and Safe Families Act, 1997, U.S., 155
affirmative action, 61
African-American families, 41–63
Aid to Dependent Children program (ADC), 44, 63
Aid to Families with Dependent Children program (AFDC), 44, 119–122, 128, 152, 167–68, 181–82
American Political Science Association, 3
Anglo-American welfare regimes, 2, 7–10, 113–35, 165–91
attentiveness as normative concept, 26
Australia, welfare in, 7, 87–109
Austria, care allowances in, 68–82
autonomy: economic, 73–74, 80; diminution of, 145–48; subconcepts of, 29–30

Baker, Maureen, 7
Bakke, Edward, 49
Baldwin, James, 41, 59
Bashevkin, Sylvia, 8–9
Bensonsmith, Dionne, 5–6
Beyond Entitlement (Mead), 57–60
Billingsly, Andrew, 52
"Black Ladies, Welfare Queens, and State Minstrels: Ideological War by Narrative Means" (Lubiano), 54–57

Blair, Tony, 8, 113–16, 127–35
block-transfer vs. cost-sharing, 120, 124, 139, 170
breadwinner model, 5–18, 90–91, 100, 104–105
"broken home" discourse, 48
Bush, George, 114, 120, 152

Canada, welfare in, 7–8, 87–109, 113–16, 123–27, 130–35, 165–91
Canada Assistance Plan (CAP), 117, 124–126, 167–69
Canada Health and Social Transfer (CHST), 95, 103, 124–28, 131–32, 169–71, 178
Cardin, Benjamin, 156–57
care: alternative policies in, 183–91; "choice" and, 6–7, 187; definition of, 19–22; ethic of, 15–16, 29–35, 27–29; paid vs. unpaid, 1, 7–9, 15–35, 118, 123, 158–60, 188–91; and poverty, 158–59; right to, 69; and work, 8–9, 69–71, 81–82
care allowances, 6–7, 67–82, 158–60, 188–91
child care, 7, 91–92, 94–96, 98–109, 116, 183–91
Child Support Act of 1991, U.K., 117
child support enforcement, 121, 148–52, 154, 177–79
Child Tax Benefit, Canada, 170–71
choice: and care, 6–7, 32–33, 78, 100, 183; freedom of, 32–33; reproductive, 143–60
Chrétien, Jean, 8, 113–16, 123–27, 130–35

citizenship: and care, 33–34; dependence and, 18, 148; economically contingent, 122–23; and entitlement, 88, 155; race in, 5–6; regimes of, 69–74, 76–80; social, 11, 69–74, 87, 114, 124–25, 133–34, 155, 165–66, 180, 183; welfare and, 6–7, 41–63, 147–48; women's, 3, 147–48
Clinton, Bill, 8, 113–23, 126, 128, 130–35, 143, 168
Code of Social and Family Responsibility, New Zealand, 101
Collins, Patricia Hill, 52
"combination scenario," 15, 18
competence as normative concept, 27
conceptual issues, 4–35
Congress, U.S., 119–20, 156–57, 168
conservative ideology, 113–17, 123–24, 166, 178–80
Conservative party, Canada, 101, 124, 130, 178
Contract with America, 120, 168

Dahrendorf, Ralf, 135
Davis, Angela, 52
debt, government, 92–93
decommodification, 1–2, 69, 184
Democratic party, U.S., 116, 119–23, 131–32, 144, 168
Denmark, care allowances in, 68–83
Department of Health and Human Services, U.S., 149–55
dependence: age-related, 67, 75–77; discourse on, 3–5, 123–24; as feminizing, 49–50; individualized, 169; on men, 16–17, 144–45; punitive solutions to, 117, 134–35; on welfare, 90–92, 95–104, 180
distributive paradigm, the, 16–35
divorce: mandatory education on, 150; rates of, 95
Domestic Purposes Benefit, New Zealand, 91
Dutch Emancipation Council, 19–21

Earned Income Tax Credit, U.S. (EITC), 119–23, 129, 132
earning levels, 92–99
elder care, 6–7, 67–82, 91
employability programs, 99–109
employer lobbies, 100–101
Employment Contracts Act of 1991, New Zealand, 103
entitlement, 88–90, 122, 155, 170, 184
equality as normative concept, 30–31, 184–85
Esping-Andersen, Gøsta, 1–4, 88, 115
ethic of care, 15–16, 23–25, 29–35

family: African-American, 42–63; and care, 69–70; internal economy of, 77–79; nuclear, 177–83; planning of, 152–53, 173–74; right to make decisions on, 9, 143–60; and state/market relations, 2–3, 91–92
Family Benefits Act of 1967, Canada, 176
family cap policies, 121, 152–53, 174–75
Family Support Act 1998, U.S., 116–17
"family values," 117, 166, 177–78, 180, 191
family wage, 90–91, 98
"fatherhood initiatives," U.S., 149–50, 156–57

fathers: as wage supplement, 156–57; rights of, 9, 48–51
female/female variations, 4
feminism: care ethic of, 15–16, 23–25; influence on policy, 98–103; and Moynihan Report, 52, 54–57; and social citizenship, 165–66; on welfare states, 1–11, 126–27, 183–91; on women's care work, 157–60
Finland, care allowances in, 68–82
Fisher, Berenice, 23–25
Food Stamps, 156, 168
foster care, 154–55
frail elderly, the, 6–7, 67–82, 91
France, care allowances in, 68–82
freedom of choice as normative concept, 32–33

gender roles: and care allowances, 68–82, 183–88; and employability programs, 99–109; and family structure, 46–51; and market relations, 6–7, 182–91; and Moynihan Report, 5, 42–63; and policy, 165, 190–91
General Welfare Assistance Act of 1958, Canada, 176
Germany, care allowances in, 67–82
Giddings, Paula, 44
globalization, 92–98
government, structure of, 102–104
Great Britain (*See*, United Kingdom)
Great Society programs, 58–61

Harman, Harriet, 128–29
Hill, Anita, 55–56

illegitimacy ratio, 144–50, 173

independence as normative concept, 19–29, 166
interest group mobilization, 98–103
International Political Science Association, 3

Jackson, Jesse, Jr., 156–58
Jencks, Christopher, 51
Jenson, Jane, 6–7
Jim Crow laws, 48
job placement, 175–76, 178–80
Johnson, Lyndon, 42, 59, 134
Johnson, Nancy, 149, 156–57

King, Mackenzie, 123

labor market, gender in, 6–7, 67–71, 87–109, 118, 180–91
Labour Party, U.K., 92–107, 114, 116, 128–30
Ladner, Joyce, 52
leave, paid: gender-specific, 185, 188–91; parental, 10, 185–88
Liberal party, Canada, 114, 116, 123–24, 130–31
"Liberal Retreat from Race during the Post-Civil Rights Era, The" (Steinberg), 53–54
lifetime limits, 170, 175–75
Lubiano, Wahneema, 52, 54–57

"man-in-the-house" rule, 177
market relations: in child care, 180–83; in elder care, 73–82; ideology of, 73; increased reliance on, 8–10; privileging of, 6–7; regulation of, 87–109; sex segregation in, 118, 182–83, 188–91
marriage: common-law, 177; dissolution of, 95; vs. obligatory work, 9, 41–44, 57, 143–44, 165–91
Marshall, T. H., 4, 71–72, 123
Martin, Emma Mae, 55
Martin, Paul, 124, 125

matriarchy, stereotypes of, 43–48, 54–57
Mead, Lawrence, 57–60
means-tested models, 114, 122
median income, former U.S. recipients, 155–56
Medicaid, 156
men: and breadwinner model, 16–18, 90–91; care by, 16–18, 189; dependency on, 16, 144–45; earnings of, 90–98; Moynihan on, 43–48, 59; and TANF, 143–60
Mettler, Suzanne, 61
Mink, Gwyndolyn, 8–9, 50, 61, 183–85
mothers: assumed domesticity of, 158–59; employability of, 87–109; poverty among, 155–58, 189–90; rights of, 143–60, 183–85; single, 113–35, 143–60, 165–91; social benefit for, 92–98, 107; stereotypes of, 43–48, 54–57; teenage, 120–21, 125, 157, 169
Moynihan, Daniel Patrick, 5, 42
Moynihan Report, 5–6, 42–63, 117, 147, 157–58
Mulroney, Brian, 113, 116–17

National Child Benefit, Canada, 126–27, 132
Negro Family, The: The Case for National Action (See, Moynihan Report)
neoconservatives, 113, 116–17
neoliberal restructuring, 8, 10, 87–109, 113–35, 166, 180–83, 191
Netherlands, care policies in, 4, 15–35, 67–82
New Deal work scheme, U.K., 92, 101, 127–30
New Democratic Party, Canada, 98

New Labour government, U.K., 98–101, 114, 127–30
New Zealand, welfare in, 7, 87–109
normative concepts, 15–35
Norplant birth control device, 153
nuclear family, institutionalization of, 178–83

Ontario Ministry of Community and Social Services, 177
Ontario Works workfare program, 8, 125, 165–66, 171–77, 180–83

parental leave, 10, 185–88
parental rights, 149–55
Parents' Fair Share program, 149
Partners for Fragile Families program, 149
Pateman, Carole, 184–85
paternity, establishment of, 120–21, 126, 131, 148–55, 172–74
patriarchal family, restoration of, 143–60
Personal Responsibility and Work Opportunity Reconciliation Act of 1996, U.S. (PRWORA), 8–9, 57, 119–23, 132, 143–44, 157–58, 168–71, 173, 178
personal responsibility discourse, 3, 5, 8–9, 16, 87, 133–35, 148, 157–58
Pierson, Paul, 1, 3, 121–22
policy: on care, 15–35; discourse on, 3–5, 113–15; feminists' influence on, 98–100; and government structure, 101–105; meaning conveyed through, 62–63; moralistic, 9, 133, 147–55, 178–82, 185; normative analysis of, 15–18; race and, 5–6, 113–35

poor: deserving vs. undeserving, 41–44; working, 101
"post-conservative" politics, 8, 113–35
poverty: and care, 156–58; as moral flaw, 117–19, 133–34; persistence among mothers, 97, 155–58, 189–90; racialized, 44–51, 146–47; tolerance for, 101; "war on," 134
power, 23–25
power resource theorists, 102
"Price of the Ticket, The" (Baldwin), 41
public/private relationship, 33–34, 71–77

race: and care, 185–86; and citizenship, 41–63; and policy, 5–6; and poverty, 44–51, 146–47; and restructuring, 106–107; and TANF, 143, 146–47; and welfare reform, 133–35
"rational man" model, 106–108
Reagan, Ronald, 8, 113, 116–17
relationality as normative concept, 26
reproductive choice, 143–60
Republican party, U.S., 117, 119–20, 131, 144, 157, 168
residual welfare state, 2, 115, 122–23
responsibility as normative concept, 26
responsiveness as normative concept, 27–28
Responsible Fatherhood Act proposed, U.S., 149–50, 156–57
retrenchment theory, 121–22
rights violations, U.S., 143–60
Royal Commission on the Status of Women, Canada, 99

sanction penalties, 154
"second earners," 92

self-sufficiency as normative concept, 19–29, 95, 106–107, 166, 176–78, 180
sexual privacy, 143–60, 177–78
Sevenhuijsen, Selma, 5, 9
slavery, 43, 45, 48
Social Assistance Reform Act of 1997, Canada, 176, 178
social citizenship, 11, 69–74, 87, 114, 124–25, 133–34, 155, 165–66, 180, 183
Social Exclusion Unit, U.K., 128
social insurance approach, 88–89
Social Security Act of 1935, U.S., 63
social security as per cent of GDP, 80
Social Union Framework Agreement, Canada (SUFA), 170, 182
Staples, Robert, 52
state, role of, 2–4, 59–62, 89–92, 186–88
state/market/family relations, 2–4
Steinberg, Stephen, 53–54
stereotypes, 43–48, 54–57
Straight from the Heart (Chrétien), 123
Sweden, gendered caregiving in, 186, 188

tax rates, 92–94
taxified/fiscalized social policy, 8, 114–16, 122–23, 128–32, 170–71
Temporary Assistance to Needy Families (TANF), 44, 120–21, 143–60, 168–71, 173, 181
Thatcher, Margaret, 8, 101, 113, 116–17
Third Way policies, 8, 78, 113–35
Thomas, Clarence, 55–56
Tory party, U.K., 8, 100, 117

"Towards a New Balance between Work and Care" (Netherlands government), 20–21, 30–31
trade unions, 97–99
Tronto, Joan, 23–25, 34
Trudeau, Pierre, 134
trust as normative concept, 28
typology of welfare states, 1–3, 88, 115

"underclass," the, 53–58
universal caregiver model, 191
United Kingdom (U.K.): care allowances in, 68–82; restructuring in, 87–109; Third Way policies in, 113–16, 127–35; welfare in, 7
United States (U.S.): early welfare in, 44, 49–51; moralistic approaches in, 9, 133, 147–55, 178–82, 185; race in, 5–6, 41–63, 133–35; violations of rights in, 143–60; welfare reform in, 113–23, 130–35, 165–91

values expressed in care policy, 24–35, 78, 113, 133–35, 185–91
vocational freedom, 143–60
Vosko, Leah F., 9–10

W-2 workfare program, 10, 165–66, 171–77, 180–83
wage: family, 91, 98; father as supplement to, 156–57; living, 108; minimum, 121; and race, 147; rates of, 92–99
"war on poverty," 134
Walker, Margaret Urban, 26–27
"welfare queen," 42–43, 54–56, 63

welfare reform, 8–10, 104–109, 113–35, 143–60
welfare state: change in, 3–11; and care, 180–91; and citizenship, 11, 60–62; feminists on, 1–11, 126–127, 183–91; literature on, 1–4, 190–91; models of, 88–92; as police state, 9, 143–60; residual, 2, 115, 122–23; and restructuring, 87–135; retrenchment of, 121–29; and single motherhood, 113–35, 143–60, 165–91; typology of, 1–3, 88, 115
Western European welfare states, 6–7, 67–82, 159
Wiley, George, 51
Wilson, William Julius, 53–54
Wisconsin, welfare reform in, 10, 165–66, 171–77, 180–83
Witteveen, Willem, 28
women: as benefit recipients, 1, 165–91; and care, 4, 6, 183–91; influence on policy, 98–103, 116–17; violations of rights of, 143–60
work: vs. benefits, 88–109; and care, 15–35, 69–74, 81, 90–109, 115, 117–18, 156–60, 188–91; vs. marriage, 41–44, 57, 143–44, 165–91; by mothers, 87–135; obligatory, 9–10; redefinition of, 182–91
workfare schemes, 9–10, 92, 94–104, 113–35, 143–60, 165–91
Working Families Tax Credit, U.K., 129, 132
workless households, 128
work-tested benefits, 115–16, 122–23, 125–27
work-training placement, 176, 181